Making Healthy Decisions
Fitness

Unit 2

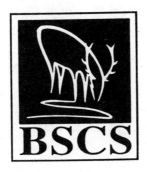

BSCS

KENDALL/HUNT PUBLISHING COMPANY

4050 Westmark Drive   Dubuque, Iowa 52002

ISBN 0-7872-1224-5

This work was supported by the Gates Foundation, the Helen K. and Arthur E. Johnson Foundation, the Piton
Foundation, and the Adolph Coors Foundation. However, the opinions expressed herein do not necessarily reflect
the position or policies of the funding agencies, and no official endorsement should be inferred.

10 9 8 7 6 5 4 3 2 1

TABLE OF CONTENTS

UNIT 2: FITNESS

FOREWORD

Whether you are aware of it or not, you make decisions about your health all day, every day. You are making decisions about your health when you decide what to eat for breakfast or whether to eat breakfast at all, whether to brush and floss your teeth, whether to wear a safety belt if you ride to school in a car, how to communicate with your classmates and teachers once you arrive at school, what to eat for lunch, whether to participate in sports or exercise after school, which television programs you watch, and when you go to sleep. Believe it or not, just about everything you do has some impact on your health and YOU are in charge of most of those decisions. Are the decisions you make healthy ones? How do you know? Do you care?

Sometimes, it's tough to make healthy decisions. All of us have lots of excuses: It's not what my friends are doing. I'm not sick, so why worry about what I eat? I'm careful, so I'm not going to get hurt. I really don't have time to exercise. No one else in the car has on a safety belt. In the lessons you are about to experience, we hope to convince you that it makes sense to pay attention to your health while you're healthy. Although some of the actions you take might not have an effect until years later, many decisions will make a difference right now in how you feel, how you relate to your friends and family, whether or not you become injured, whether you contract a life-threatening illness, or whether you put someone else's life and health at risk.

We sincerely hope you enjoy the activities in this unit of *Making Healthy Decisions* and that they make a difference in how you care for yourself and those around you. Remember, the healthy decisions are up to you.

Nancy M. Landes
Revision Director

James D. Ellis
Project Director
Field-test Edition

INTRODUCTION TO FITNESS

What does physical fitness mean to you? According to the President's Council on Physical Fitness and Sports, a fit person is one who:

has the energy and strength to perform daily activities vigorously and alertly without getting "run down," and

has energy left over to enjoy leisure-time activities and meet emergency demands.

Do you meet those guidelines? Do you participate in some type of vigorous physical activity, such as brisk walking, jogging, swimming, basketball, or soccer, at least three times a week?

Being fit can be fun for everyone. You don't have to be an athlete or be "the best" to become fit, but you do have to be active and participate in some form of physical activity at least three times a week. Through the lessons in this unit, you will experience the benefits of fitness and determine your current level of fitness. By working out with your classmates, you can improve your level of fitness and have fun at the same time. Becoming physically fit doesn't require special skills or athletic abilities. YOU can do it!

Personal health is not something you can take for granted. Investing in fitness is one way to gain big health benefits, both now and in the future. Not only will you look better as you "shape up," but you will feel great and have more energy to enjoy the things you like to do.

Becoming more active is a healthy decision you can make. Get up off that couch, turn off the TV, and get moving. It's up to you to make fitness fun!

FINDING OUT ABOUT FITNESS

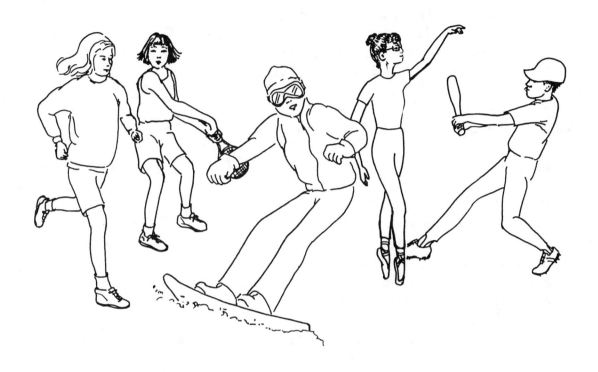

Being physically fit means having the energy and strength to perform daily activities vigorously and alertly without getting "run down," and to have energy left over to enjoy leisure-time activities or meet emergency demands. When you are physically fit, your heart, lungs, and muscles are strong and your body is firm and flexible. Your weight and percent body fat are within a desirable range.

Physical fitness will help you control your weight and cope with stress. You'll feel and look better, and that often means success in anything you want to do, such as work, sports, dance, and other recreational activities. You may even do better in school.

Getting in shape is important for your future. You'll be healthier both now and as an adult, and that means a more enjoyable and active life.*

*Source: President's Council on Physical Fitness and Sports. *Get Fit!* (1993). Bloomington, IN: President's Challenge, p. 6.

Stop and Discuss

What do you know and believe about physical fitness? Discuss the following questions about the who, what, when, and why of fitness.

1. Who should be involved in physical fitness?
2. What should they do to become physically fit?
3. When, and for how long, should they be involved in fitness activities?
4. Why should they be involved in physical fitness?

ACTIVITY: TAKING A FITNESS SURVEY

Procedure

1. Review BLM 1.1, A Fitness Survey.
2. Complete one survey yourself.
3. Take two surveys home and ask two friends or family members each to complete one. Bring the completed surveys to class.
   Survey people of various ages. Also, survey people who have differing opinions or actions regarding physical fitness.
4. Report the survey results on chart paper.
   Divide the paper into two columns and report the answers from regular exercisers on one side and the answers from nonexercisers on the other.
5. Compare your answers on the fitness survey (from Step 2) with those listed on the chart.
6. As a class, discuss your reactions to the survey results.

ACTIVITY: WORKING OUT

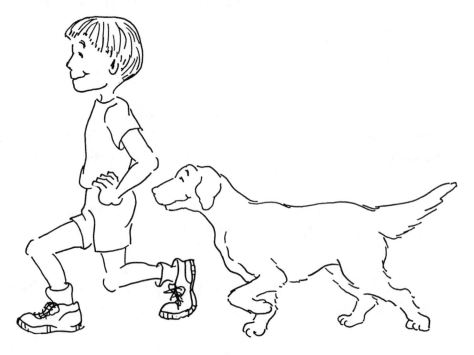

Your teacher will lead you in a fitness workout. As you go through the activities and exercises, pay attention to how you feel before, during, and after each part of the workout. After the workout, think about your level of physical fitness. Are you as fit as you would like to be?

WRAP UP

Look at people's answers to question 4f on the survey: What would motivate you to be more physically active? Use those suggestions and the answers to question 5 and brainstorm a fitness event that might motivate you, your classmates, and family members to find fitness fun. Your teacher has a form that will help you plan the who, what, when, and why of a fun fitness event.

The following are some ideas: sponsor a walk-a-thon or a bike-a-thon for a worthy cause, conduct morning exercises over the PA (public address) system at school, lead after-school exercises or activities at a nearby elementary school, have a field day, participate in "jump rope for heart," or have all-school relays. Use your imagination!

INVOLVING FAMILY MEMBERS

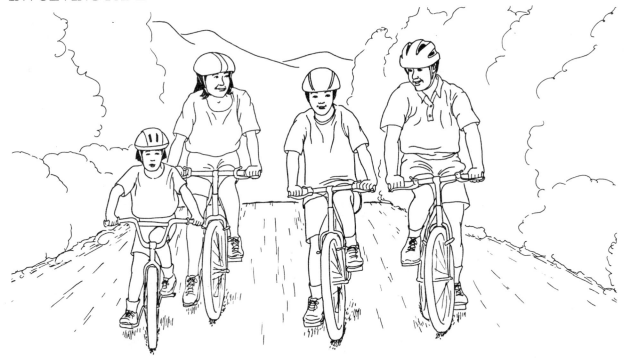

Physical fitness is a fun reason for your family to do things together. After every lesson in this unit, there will be suggestions for involving family members in your fitness efforts. Because fitness is not something you can develop just during school hours, you need to think about fun ways to get your friends and family involved. It will help you and them live a healthier life.

Ask your family members to complete the fitness survey at home. How many of them exercise regularly? If they do, what reasons do they give for exercising? If they do not, what reasons do they give for not exercising? As a family, plan one activity that you could do together that would promote physical fitness. It could be a bike ride, a walk after dinner, or a basketball game. Choose something that everyone can enjoy.

ON TARGET

READING: CARDIOVASCULAR FITNESS

No one can say *exactly* how fit each of us should be, but experts know that overall fitness is a combination of many things, including

- exercising regularly,
- maintaining moderate weight,
- eating breakfast,
- eating well-balanced meals,
- not snacking between meals,
- avoid smoking, and
- sleeping at least seven to eight hours each night.

In this unit, you will be looking mainly at the relationship between exercise and physical fitness. You will learn about five components of physical fitness: cardiovascular fitness, muscular strength, muscular endurance, flexibility, and body composition. Each is developed by different activities and exercises.

This lesson deals with the first of the components—cardiovascular fitness. Cardiovascular fitness can be defined as the measure of how well your muscles can continue activities for a sustained period of time. It also refers to the ability of the heart, blood, and blood vessels (arteries, veins, and capillaries) to transport oxygen to all body cells, especially to the muscle cells, and to carry away waste products. The term "cardio" refers to the heart; the term "vascular" refers to the blood vessels. The terms "cardiorespiratory fitness" (cardio = heart, respiratory = the lungs and other parts of the respiratory system) and "aerobic fitness" (activities requiring high levels of oxygen) are other terms for the same type of fitness.

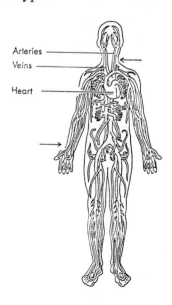

Arteries

Veins

Heart

A person who has achieved cardiovascular fitness has a very efficient blood-pumping system. Because the heart is a muscle, it can actually grow larger and stronger when it is exercised regularly. A fit heart is a more efficient heart--it can do its job with less effort. (You will explore this idea further in the activity "How Does Cardiovascular Fitness Affect Your Heart?") When you have cardiovascular fitness, you will not get out of breath as quickly as you would if you were not fit. Having a fit heart reduces a person's chances of having heart attacks and strokes—two major killers of adults. Aerobic exercise—exercise that builds cardiovascular endurance—also helps control the amount of fat on a person's body. Aerobic exercise uses a lot of energy.

Activities that improve cardiovascular fitness include running, swimming, bicycling, cross-country skiing, jumping rope, and aerobic dancing. These are considered "aerobic" activities because they require the body to use high levels of oxygen. To improve cardiovascular fitness, aerobic exercise should last at least 15 minutes without stopping. To keep fit, a person should do some type of aerobic activity at least three times a week.

So, how can you get your heart in better shape? The best way is to exercise at your **target heart rate** three or four times a week for 15-20 minutes each time. The target heart rate is the rate at which your heart should be beating during exercise to get the greatest benefit from that exercise. If you exercise above that rate, you are working your heart too hard. Below that rate, your heart is not working hard enough to become stronger.

To measure your target heart rate, you have to know how to measure your heart rate. You measure your heart rate by taking your pulse. If you are not sure how to take your pulse, complete the next activity. If you already know how to take your pulse accurately, then go to the next activity "Finding My Target Heart Rate."

ACTIVITY: TAKING MY PULSE

Every time your heart muscles contract, your heart pumps blood through your body. Blood travels through the blood vessels to all parts of your body. Arteries carry blood from your heart through your body, and veins carry the blood from your body back to your heart.

Some of your arteries are near the surface of the skin where you can feel the blood pulsing through them. Each time you feel a pulse, or a beat, your heart has contracted. The number of times your artery pulses in one minute is called your **pulse rate**. Your pulse rate is the same as your heart rate.

When you exercise to improve cardiovascular fitness, you will need to measure your exercising pulse rate. Follow the procedure and learn to measure your pulse rate as accurately as possible.

Procedure

1.   Look at the following photographs that show two ways you can measure your pulse. *Notice that you can measure your pulse at either your wrist or at the side of your neck.*

2.   Because the pulse in the side of the neck is stronger and easier to find, try that first. Place the flat part of two fingers in the hollow spot at the side of your neck, just under your chin and above your Adam's apple. Press in lightly.

You can use your right hand to feel a pulse on the right side of your neck or your left hand to feel a pulse on the left side of your neck. Be sure to use your fingertips and not your thumb to find your pulse. Your thumb has a tiny pulse of its own and might confuse your counting. Don't press too hard. If you can't feel your pulse right away, move your fingers around on that part of your neck until you feel a slight "jump" in the artery.

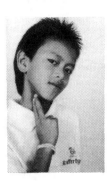

3.   Count your pulse for 15 seconds.
Either have someone else time for you, or watch the second hand on a clock.

4.   Multiply your pulse by 4 or use the Heart-Rate Chart to determine the number of pulses or beats per minute.
Usually, exercising and resting pulses are measured in beats per minute; however, you don't have to count for 60 seconds to get an accurate reading.

5.   Now, try to find your pulse at your wrist. Place the flat part of two fingers of one hand on the thumb side of your other wrist as shown in the following photograph. Feel between the bones and above the wrist joint. Press in lightly.

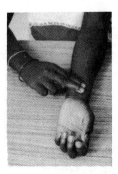

6.   To practice, take your pulse a few different times.
Try taking your pulse at your wrist and at the side of your neck. Do you get a similar pulse rate each time?

7.   With a partner, practice taking one another's pulse.

You might take your pulse at the side of your neck while your partner takes your pulse at your other wrist. Then, compare numbers. Did you get the same number of beats in 15 seconds? If not, practice until you do. Then take your partner's pulse in the same way. Remember, your pulse rate probably will not be the same as your partner's, but you should be able to agree on each person's pulse rate.

8.   When you exercise, you need to be able to find your pulse quickly. Practice until you can find your pulse within 2 to 3 seconds.

ACTIVITY: FINDING MY TARGET HEART RATE

During aerobic exercises, if your pulse rate does not go up enough, your heart will not become more fit. If your pulse rate is too high, your heart is working too hard. That could be dangerous. The ideal pulse rate for a person who is doing aerobic exercises is called the **target heart rate**.

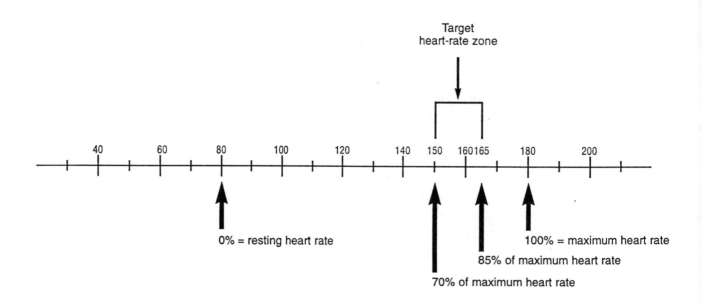

[This is a continuum for a 40-year-old person whose resting heart rate is 80 beats per minute. This indicates the difference between the person's resting heart rate and maximum heart rate, showing where 70 percent and 85 percent would fall along the continuum.]*

Your target heart rate is really a target heart-rate zone with 70 percent of your maximum heart rate as the low number and 85 percent of your maximum heart rate as the high number. Follow the procedures and calculate your target heart-rate zone. (If you have a heart problem, talk to your doctor. Find out how much you can safely exercise your heart.)

*Source: Getchell, Bud. (1983). *Physical Fitness: A Way of Life*, third edition. New York, New York: John Wiley & Sons

Procedure

1. First, find your maximum heart rate (in beats per minute) by subtracting your age from the number 220. Write that number at the top of a sheet of paper.
    For example, Monique is 13 years old. Her maximum heart rate is 220 - 13 = 207 beats per minute. That is as fast as her heart can beat. She should not make her heart work that hard for very long.

2. Multiply your maximum heart rate from Step 1 by 70 percent. Write that number at the left side of your paper.
    That number is the low side of your target heart-rate zone. In Monique's example, her low number will be 70 percent of 207 (207 X .70 = 144.9), which can be rounded off to 145 beats per minute.

3. Next, multiply your maximum heart rate from Step 1 by 85 percent. Write that number at the right side of your paper.
    That number is the high side of your target heart rate zone. In Monique's example, her high number will be 85 percent of 207 (207 X .85 = 175.9), which can be rounded off to 176 beats per minute.

4. Divide the two numbers of your target heart rate zone by 4 to find the number of beats you should count in 15 seconds if you are in your zone. (Or, you can use the Heart-Rate Chart. Remember, 15 seconds is one-fourth of one minute.)
    Monique would divide 145 and 176 beats per minute by 4 to get the number of beats in 15 seconds. (145÷4 = 36; 176÷4 = 44) This means she should count somewhere between 36 and 44 beats in 15 seconds if she is in her zone.

5. After you have calculated your target heart rate zone and know the number of beats you should count in 15 seconds, try some aerobic exercises, such as running in place or jumping jacks, for a minute or two. Take your pulse for 15 seconds after exercising and find out if you are in your zone.
    If your heart beats more times that your high number, then you are working too hard and you should slow down. If your heart beats fewer times than your low number, then you are not working hard enough and should try to speed up a little.

6. Practice as you exercise. Stop and check your pulse rate once in a while during aerobic exercise. Count the beats for only 15 seconds to avoid stopping for very long. Are you exercising within your zone?
    Concentrate on how you feel--your breathing rate, your heart beat, the tightness of your muscles--when you exercise within your target zone. After you exercise in your target zone for a period of time, you will know what it feels like, and you can monitor your exercising pace without always measuring your pulse.

ACTIVITY: HOW DOES CARDIOVASCULAR FITNESS AFFECT YOUR HEART?

When people participate regularly in aerobic exercises, their bodies change. Examples of activities that can cause body changes include cross-county skiing, distance swimming, distance walking, running, and cycling. Some changes, such as the loss of fat, are easy to observe. Other changes, such as emotional changes or a stronger heart, are not as easy to observe.

When a person's heart becomes more fit, it can pump more blood each time it contracts. The amount of blood the heart can pump in one beat is called the stroke volume. The following bar graph shows the difference in stroke volume between people who regularly do aerobic exercises and those who do not. Whose heart can pump more blood in one beat—a regular aerobic exerciser or a nonexerciser? Do you think this changes how often a person's heart must beat each day?

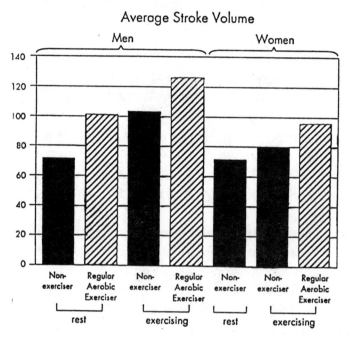

Average Stroke Volume

Procedure

1. Look at the bar graph of resting pulse rates that follows. Write the number of beats per minute for the nonexerciser and the regular aerobic exerciser.

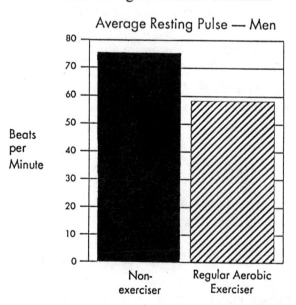

Average Resting Pulse — Men

2. Calculate how many times each person's heart beats in one day. Write the number of beats in one day for each person--the nonexerciser and the regular exerciser.
    Hint: The rates shown are in beats per minute. There are 60 minutes in one hour and 24 hours in one day.

3.   Whose heart beats more often, the nonexerciser's heart or the regular aerobic exerciser's heart? What is the difference in beats per day between the nonexerciser and the regular exerciser? What would be the difference in beats per year?

Stop and Discuss

1.   Look at the bar graph of the average stroke volume. Whose heart pumps more blood with each beat—the nonexerciser's or the regular exerciser's?
2.   Whose heart beats less often—the nonexerciser's or the regular exerciser's?
3.   Whose heart does not have to work as hard each day—the exerciser's or the nonexerciser's? (In other words, whose heart is more efficient?)
4.   Whose heart do you think is healthier? Why do you think so?

WRAP UP

Discuss answers to the following questions.

1.   What is cardiovascular fitness?
2.   How would regularly exercising your heart benefit you?
3.   Do you want to improve the fitness of your heart and lungs? Why or why not?
4.   What can you do to improve your cardiovascular fitness?

INVOLVING FAMILY MEMBERS

Teach your family members how to take their pulse and to calculate their target heart-rate zones. (Remember, younger family members will have higher numbers in their target heart-rate zones and older family members will have lower numbers.) Explain how the zone helps them decide how hard to exercise. Then, participate in some aerobic activity such as basketball, jogging, fast walking, or aerobic dancing to music and measure pulse rates during the activity. Can everyone exercise within his or her target heart-rate zone?

LESSON 3

MEASURING FITNESS

Before you begin any exercise or activity program to improve your physical fitness, it is important for you to know your starting point. How fit are you now? How fit would you like to be? The purpose of fitness testing is <u>not</u> to compare your level of fitness with someone else's. The purpose of testing is to give you a starting point from which you can measure your own improvement. Each person is unique and has a different physical make-up and history. Your results are for your own use. You do not need to share them with anyone else, but you need to know where you are now so you can plan what you need to do to become more physically fit.

Be sure you have on comfortable clothes and proper shoes for exercising. Get yourself psyched up for measuring fitness. Ready, set, go for it!

ACTIVITY: HOW FIT ARE YOU?

Procedure

1. Find a partner. Get a pencil and a record page, titled My Results Record Page, from your teacher.
   You will need a partner to complete most of the fitness tasks. Your partner will keep track of the time for each task, count the number of sit-ups or chin-ups, hold your ankles, read the measurement for the sit-and-reach task, and offer general encouragement. Choose a partner with whom you feel comfortable. Each of you will record your results on your own record page.
2. Follow your teacher's directions for completing each fitness task.
   You will complete such fitness tasks as the mile run, bent-knee sit-ups, chin-ups, and a sit-and-reach task. Your teacher will tell you where and when to do the tasks. Warm up before you complete each task.
3. After you complete each task, record the time, number, or distance on My Results Record Page in the appropriate space.
   Complete all of the fitness tasks before going on to Step 4.
4. Look at the tables that follow. In each table, locate the column for your gender (boy or girl) and age. Find your results in that column. On your record page, write the rating—Keep Up the Good Work, Doing OK, or Improvement Is Possible—that corresponds with your results.
5. Complete the first sentence on the record page under the heading, Moving On.
   Select the one area that you would most like to improve. Although you might want to improve in all areas, pick the one that is most important to you right now. You will be more likely to be successful if you don't try to fix everything all at once.

Rating Tables for Fitness Task Results

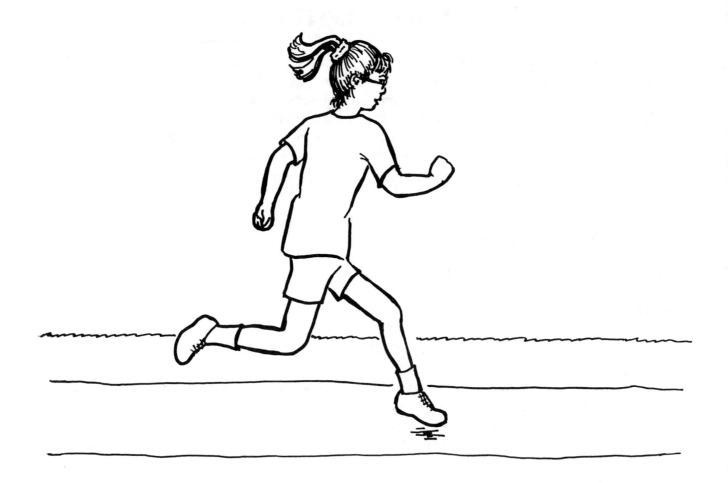

MILE RUN CHART (IN MINUTES AND SECONDS)

	BOYS (BY AGE)					GIRLS (BY AGE)				
Rating	10	11	12	13	14	10	11	12	13	14
Keep up the good work	Less than 9:02	Less than 8:12	Less than 8:03	Less than 7:24	Less than 7:18	Less than 10:27	Less than 10:10	Less than 10:05	Less than 9:48	Less than 9:31
Doing OK	9:02 to 11:00	8:12 to 10:32	8:03 to 10:13	7:24 to 9:10	7:18 to 9:06	10:27 to 12:52	10:10 to 12:54	10:05 to 12:33	9:48 to 12:17	9:31 to 11:49
Improvement is possible	More than 11:00	More than 10:32	More than 10:13	More than 9:10	More than 9:06	More than 12:52	More than 12:54	More than 12:33	More than 12:17	More than 11:49

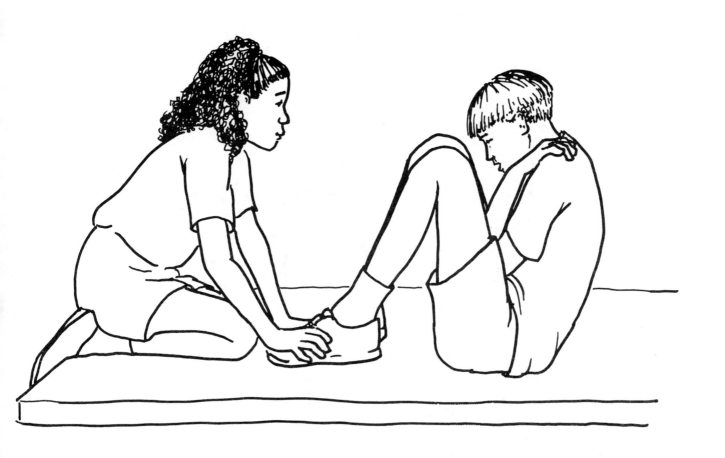

SIT-UPS CHART (NUMBER COMPLETED)

	BOYS (BY AGE)					GIRLS (BY AGE)				
Rating	10	11	12	13	14	10	11	12	13	14
Keep up the good work	More than 38	More than 40	More than 43	More than 45	More than 45	More than 36	More than 36	More than 39	More than 39	More than 40
Doing OK	28 to 38	30 to 40	32 to 43	32 to 45	35 to 45	25 to 36	26 to 36	27 to 39	28 to 39	29 to 40
Improvement is possible	Less than 28	Less than 30	Less than 32	Less than 32	Less than 35	Less than 25	Less than 26	Less than 27	Less than 28	Less than 29

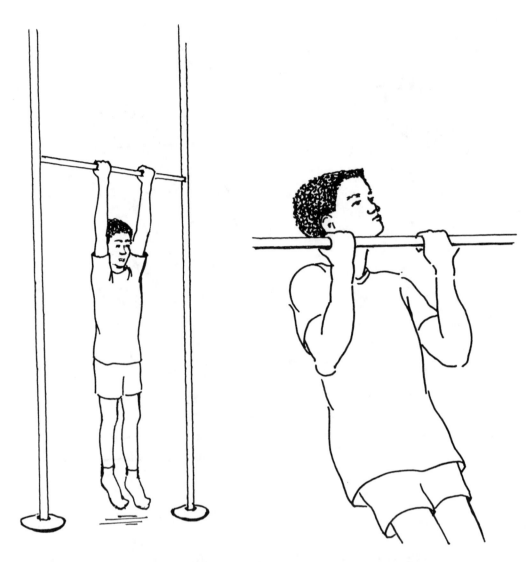

CHIN-UPS CHART (NUMBER COMPLETED)

Rating	BOYS (BY AGE)					GIRLS (BY AGE)				
	10	11	12	13	14	10	11	12	13	14
Keep up the good work	More than 4	More than 4	More than 5	More than 7	More than 8	More than 1	More than 1	More than 1	More than 1	More than 1
Doing OK	1 to 4	1 to 4	1 to 5	1 to 7	2 to 8	1	1	1	1	1
Improvement is possible	Less than 1	Less than 1	Less than 1	Less than 1	Less than 2	Less than 1	Less than 1	Less than 1	Less than 1	Less than 1

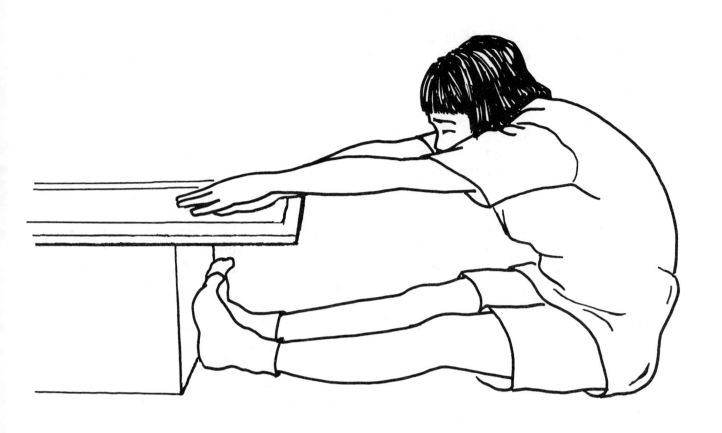

SIT-AND-REACH CHART (IN INCHES)

	BOYS (BY AGE)					GIRLS (BY AGE)				
Rating	10	11	12	13	14	10	11	12	13	14
Keep up the good work	More than 14.5	More than 14.5	More than 14.5	More than 14.5	More than 15.0	More than 16.0	More than 16.5	More than 17.0	More than 17.5	More than 18.0
Doing OK	11.5 to 14.5	11.5 to 14.5	11.0 to 14.5	11.0 to 14.5	11.0 to 15.0	13.0 to 16.0	13.0 to 16.5	14.0 to 17.0	14.0 to 17.5	15.0 to 18.0
Improvement is possible	Less than 11.5	Less than 11.5	Less than 11.0	Less than 11.0	Less than 11.0	Less than 13.0	Less than 13.0	Less than 14.0	Less than 14.0	Less than 15.0

WRAP UP

With your classmates, brainstorm ways you could improve all areas of fitness. What exercises or activities might you do to get your chin over the chin-up bar more times? What might get you in shape to run the mile in less time? How often do you think you might need to do these exercises or activities? Over what period of time?

Use the results from your brainstorming session and complete the second sentence on your record page: I can improve my performance by _____. You can list many ways to improve your performance in the area you chose, but write only those activities or exercises that you are likely to do.

Don't be discouraged if you are disappointed with your results. Most of us would like to be more physically fit, but you can only start from where you are. Now, you have the chance to work hard so that you will do better next time. Just like most things that are worth having, physical fitness takes time and perseverance. It won't happen overnight, but it <u>will</u> happen if you stick with it.

INVOLVING FAMILY MEMBERS

Measure the levels of fitness of your family members. Have family members complete the same fitness tasks you did in class. Make sure everyone warms up ahead of time and does not overdo it. (Do not have very young brothers and sisters do exactly the same tasks. They should not try to run a mile, for example, and they might not be able to do chin-ups or sit-ups. You can think up simple tasks for them to do, such as running back and forth between two chairs a few times, and using their arms to push themselves up from the floor.) Choose one or two areas of fitness to work on as a family. Plan some fun activities you could do a few times a week that would improve your fitness, too.

LESSON 4

CALORIES DO COUNT

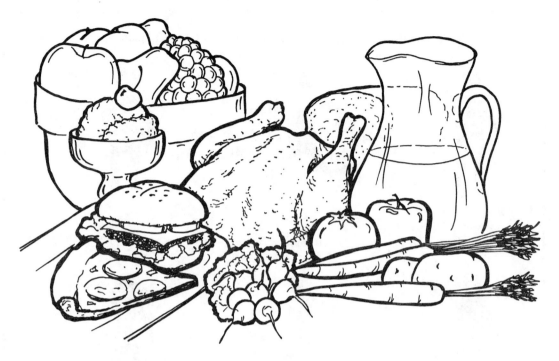

READING: WHAT ARE CALORIES?

Every minute of every day, you are burning calories. You have to have calories to survive and to perform even the most basic activities. You get your calories from the food you eat. All foods and drinks (except water) have calories. Some have a lot of calories, others have very few. You can count the calories you take in by looking in books that list the number of calories in the foods you eat. You also can count the calories you use by keeping track of all your activities and by estimating your basal (resting) metabolic rate (BMR), which is the number of calories you burn to maintain body functions. You will learn about your basal metabolic rate later.

What is a calorie? Technically, a calorie is the amount of heat it takes to raise the temperature of one gram of water one degree Celsius. All you really need to know to maintain a calorie balance is that calories are measures of energy and that energy is stored in food. You get the stored energy (calories) by eating and digesting food. Your body then "burns" or uses those food calories during all your daily activities. All the calories you take in are available for you as energy. If you don't use them, they are stored for later use. Unused calories are stored in your body as—you guessed it—fat.

You need calories for everything you do, from sleeping to running. Some general rules to remember about calories are

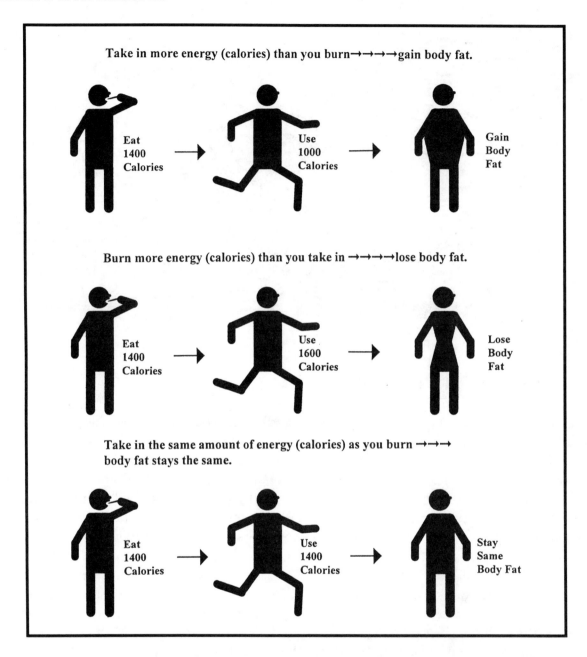

Your need for calories is changing constantly, depending on your age, your weight, your level of activity, whether or not you are still growing, and a number of other factors.

In this lesson, you will learn how to keep track of the calories you are using or burning. The nice thing about burning calories through activity is that the more you burn, the more you can eat in return! One caution, though. You need to replace the calories you burn with good, nutritious calories that will also replace the protein, carbohydrates, vitamins, minerals, and essential fats that your body uses. (The lessons in the nutrition units of *Making Healthy Decisions* will give you information about choosing a healthy diet.)

ACTIVITY: ESTIMATING YOUR DAILY CALORIE REQUIREMENTS

Did you know that you burn a certain number of calories every hour of every day, even when you are doing "nothing"? Those calories make it possible for all of your organs to work, for your brain to function, for your cells to be repaired, for injuries to be healed, and for bones and muscles to grow.

The number of calories burned to maintain body functions is called your basal (resting) metabolic rate, or BMR. You can get a rough estimate of your BMR by completing this activity. Remember, this is a very rough estimate. Determining your exact BMR would take some very sophisticated computer equipment and a very specialized person to do the testing.

You can estimate your BMR by determining the number of calories you would burn if you did nothing for 24 hours each day. This will measure the number of calories your body needs to take care of its basic needs like breathing, cell repair, circulation of blood, sending nerve impulses, growing, and other functions. Remember that this is only an estimate.

Then, you can estimate your daily need for calories by adding your BMR and your level of activity. The more active you are, the more calories you can consume and not gain weight or body fat. If you like to eat, it pays to think FITNESS!

Procedure

1. Review the information on the chart that follows. Using this information, calculate the number of calories you would need if you did nothing for 24 hours. Write the number of calories on a piece of paper and label it "My BMR Estimate."
    This is an estimate of your basal metabolic rate (BMR), the number of calories your body needs every day just to function.

Weight in Pounds	Calories Burned Per Hour	Weight in Pounds	Calories Burned Per Hour
71 or less	35	127 - 137	60
72 - 82	40	138 - 148	60
83 - 93	45	149 - 159	65
94 - 104	50	160 - 170	70
105 - 115	50	171 - 181	75
116 - 126	55	182 or more	80

2. Now you need to estimate your level of activity. You have three choices: not very active, moderately active, very active. Choose one of the three categories and write it next to your BMR estimate from Step 1.
3. If you chose the category "not very active," multiply your BMR estimate from Step 1 by 40 percent. If you chose the category "moderately active," multiply your BMR estimate from Step 1 by 60 percent. If you chose the category "very active," multiply your BMR estimate from Step 1 by 80 percent. Write that number and label it "Activity Calories."

4. Add the number of calories from Step 1, your BMR estimate, to the number of calories from Step 3, your "activity calories." This sum is an estimate of the calories you need each day to maintain your level of activity.

    Generally, males ages 11-18 need between 2,700 and 2,800 calories a day and females of the same ages need between 2,100 and 2,200 calories. (The range can be from 2,000 to 3,900 calories for males depending on the level of activity and from 1,200 to 3,000 calories for females.) The following things affect your BMR:

    - *Your gender. The BMR for males is slightly higher than for females. This is because men are usually larger and have more lean body mass than females at a given age.*
    - *Your weight. The more you weigh, the higher your BMR because your body has to work harder to carry itself around.*
    - *Your age. As you age, your BMR gets lower. This is usually because the amount of lean muscle tissue decreases and the amount of fat increases.*
    - *Your level of body fat. Lean muscle tissue uses more calories than fat tissue, even when the muscles aren't "working." Therefore, if you have more fat and less muscle, you don't need as many calories to maintain your weight.*
    - *How much you sleep. Your BMR is about 10 percent lower when you sleep.*
    - *The temperature. Colder temperatures mean your body must work harder to maintain its core temperature of 98.6 degrees F.*

Stop and Discuss

1. Explain the term "basal metabolic rate" (BMR) in your own words. How could you increase your BMR?
2. Do you think you maintain a balance between the number of calories you use and the number of calories you consume? Why or why not?
3. If you are not satisfied with your weight or percent body fat, what healthy choices could you make to change them?
4. Discuss the issue of "body image." What influences your feelings about your body image?

READING: BODY COMPOSITION

Everyone's body is composed of lean body mass and fat. Your lean body mass is made up of your body's organs, such as the heart, lungs, and liver, your bones, and your muscles. Whatever is not lean body tissue is body fat. Everyone needs some body fat for warmth, for padding of essential organs, and for energy reserves. But, many of us have too much body fat compared to our lean body mass.

One of the problems in our present-day society is that we live a sedentary, or a "sitting," lifestyle. We spend many hours sitting at computer terminals, sitting at a desk, sitting in a car or on public transportation, sitting in front of the television, or sitting with video games. Body fat loves sitting. The more we sit, the more body fat we get.

Weight does not always reveal a person's level of body fat. Sometimes, people look thin and have "normal" weight according to height/weight charts, but they can still have high levels of body fat. Some people can be above their "normal" weight on the charts and still have a low level of body fat. Those people who develop their lean body mass, especially their muscle tone, might weigh more but are actually heathier than those who look thin but have high body fat levels. Skinfold measurements can help you determine your level of body fat compared with your lean body mass.

What are the dangers of having too much body fat? Too much body fat can lead to cardiovascular disease because your heart and lungs work harder than they need to and often the arteries leading to the heart become clogged with fatty deposits. High levels of body fat also lead to high blood pressure, kidney disease, and strokes. High body fat can increase the risk of heart attacks, blood clots, varicose veins, gout, respiratory diseases, stomach and intestinal disorders, liver disease, and arthritis. Those problems usually don't show up during the teenage years, however. The main problems with excess body fat in the teen years are self-image, ability and desire to be active and have fun, lack of muscle tone, and a lack of energy.

If your level of body fat is not what you would like it to be, what can you do? One of the worst things you can do is to go on a diet. Many teens turn to fad diets, diet pills, laxatives, and appetite suppressants if they don't feel good about their body image. Those remedies can be harmful, especially because teenagers are still growing and changing. Many experts recommend that you "grow into your weight." That means that you maintain your weight and try to stop any weight gain, but the goal is not to lose weight, or at least not a lot of weight. The goal is to lose fat and increase your lean body mass by eating nutritious foods and becoming more active, not by starving yourself. When you increase your lean body mass by improving your muscle tone, you will automatically burn more calories because lean body mass requires more calories to maintain itself than does fat. Remember your BMR? With a higher percentage of lean body mass, your BMR goes up and you burn more calories even when you are doing "nothing." That's another great benefit of getting fit!

When you think about your body image, the important thing to remember is that everyone's body is different. We all inherit a basic body shape and our ultimate height. We cannot do a lot about those things, but we can take care of ourselves, make the most of what we have, and appreciate our differences. Chris Silkwood and Nancy Levicki, authors of *Awesome Teen*, say it this way:

> Teens are generally encouraged to be achievers...shoot for the moon, go after your dream. Great words, but when dealing with your physical self, some limitations can and do exist. This is why a realistic image is so important. Limitations are simply a part of being a unique human being. It is what allows one person to look very different from the next and makes life so interesting. It sure would be boring if you and all your friends looked exactly alike, dressed the very same way and had the same hairstyles. The perfect body isn't the one that fits easily into the size 4 jeans. The perfect body is one that is full of energy, stands with confident posture, is well groomed, has a self assured stride with head up high and a terrific smile.

Caring about yourself by finding ways to become more active is one key to success.

WRAP UP

Use the two charts—Food Chart and Activity Chart—and compare your "calories in" and "calories out. Are you in balance? First, from the Food Chart select a day's menu including breakfast, lunch, dinner, and snacks. Choose foods that you would actually eat and drink. If your favorite foods are not on the list, find the closest substitutes. Don't forget to include the butter, margarine, or jelly you put on your toast, the extra sugar you might add to your bowl of cereal, or the soft drink you have after school. Add up the calories you would take in if you ate those foods. (Be sure to pay attention to the serving sizes, too.)

Next, from the Activity Chart, select activities that you like to do. Then, calculate how much time you would need to spend at those various activities to balance your calorie intake from the Food Chart. Remember to add your BMR estimate to the "activity calories" from the chart. Are you active enough to keep your calories in balance?

INVOLVING FAMILY MEMBERS

Take this little quiz with your family members. It should make you think about your eating patterns and habits. After you take the quiz, talk about what you might do to change your eating patterns to be more healthy. Discuss how you might be more active as a family and burn up some of those extra calories.

1. What do I usually eat?
   Lots of fruits and vegetables
   Deep-fat-fried and breaded foods
   "Extras," such as salad dressings, potato toppings, spreads, sauces, and gravies
   Sweets and rich desserts, such as candy, cakes, and pies
   Snack foods high in fat and sodium, such as chips and other "munchies"

2. How much of the above foods do I usually eat?
   A single small serving
   A large serving
   Two servings or more

3. When do I usually eat?
   At mealtime only
   While preparing meals or clearing the table
   While watching TV or participating in other activities
   At coffee breaks
   Anytime

4. Where do I usually eat?
   At the kitchen or dining room table
   At restaurants or fast-food places
   At my desk
   In front of the TV or while reading
   Wherever I happen to be when I'm hungry

5. Why do I usually eat?
   Because it's time to eat
   Because I'm hungry
   Because foods look tempting
   Because everyone else is eating
   Because food will get thrown away if I don't eat it
   Because I'm bored, frustrated, nervous, or sad

FOOD CHART

Sugar and fat notes: "Fatty" means the food has a lot of fat. "Some fat" means the food has a medium amount of fat. "Low fat" means the food has a little fat. "Sugary" means the food has a lot of sugar. "Some sugar" means the food has a medium amount of sugar. "Low sugar" means the food has a little sugar, often natural sugar such as that in fruits. If there is no note about sugar or fat, the food has little or no fat or sugar.

Food	Number of Calories in 1 Serving
Dairy Products	
Milk (whole)	160 calories in 1 cup (fatty)
Milk (skim)	90 calories in 1 cup (low fat)
Chocolate milk (2%)	190 calories in 1 cup (some fat)
Cottage cheese	260 calories in 1 cup (low fat)
Ice cream	95 calories in 1 scoop (3 oz.) (fatty)
Butter pecan ice cream	320 calories in 4 ounces (fatty)
Chocolate ice cream	280 calories in 4 ounces (fatty)
Strawberry ice cream	260 calories in 4 ounces (fatty)
Vanilla ice cream	280 calories in 4 ounces (fatty)
Plain yogurt	125 calories in 1 cup (low fat)
Cream cheese	120 calories in 1 ounce (fatty)
Cheddar cheese	115 calories in 1 ounce (fatty)
American cheese	105 calories in 1 ounce (low fat)
Mozzarella cheese	95 calories in 1 ounce (low fat)
Parmesan cheese	100 calories in 1 ounce (fatty)
Swiss cheese	110 calories in 1 ounce (fatty)
Meat & Eggs	
Egg (boiled)	85 calories in 1 large (cholesterol)
Bacon	90 calories in two slices (fatty)
Pot roast of beef	254 calories in 3 ounces (some fat)
Corned beef	350 calories in 4 ounces (some fat)
Steak	330 calories in 3 ounces (some fat)

Beef stew	210 calories in 1 cup (some fat)
Chili (with beans)	335 calories in 1 cup (some fat)
Roast lamb	235 calories in 3 ounces (some fat)
Ham	245 calories in 3 ounces (some fat)
Ham (canned)	140 calories in 4 ounces (fatty)
Pepperoni	270 calories in 2 ounces (fatty)
Pork chop	260 calories in 1 thick chop (some fat)
Bologna	80 calories in 2 slices (fatty)
Hamburger (just the meat)	245 calories in 1 patty (fatty)
Hot dog	170 calories in 1 (fatty)
Fried chicken drumstick	90 calories in 1 (some fat)
Fried chicken breast	155 calories in 1 (some fat)
Turkey (roasted)	135 calories in 4 ounces (some fat)
Chicken (roasted)	190 calories in 4 ounces (some fat)
Flounder (baked)	220 calories in 4 ounces (low fat)
Haddock (broiled)	150 calories in 4 ounces (low fat)
Halibut (broiled)	200 calories in 4 ounces (low fat)
Salmon (steamed)	225 calories in 4 ounces (low fat)
Tuna (fresh, raw)	155 calories in 4 ounces
Tuna (canned, in water)	120 calories in 4 ounces (low fat)
Tuna (canned, in oil)	500 calories in 4 ounces (fatty)
Fish sticks	80 calories in 2 (some fat)
Crabmeat	85 calories in 3 ounces (low fat)
Shrimp	100 calories in 3 ounces (low fat)
Beans & Peanuts	
Beans (pinto, navy, cooked)	200 calories in 1 cup (low fat)
Peanuts	840 calories in 1 cup (fatty)
Peanut butter	95 calories in 1 tablespoon (fatty)

Vegetables	
Asparagus	10 calories in 4 pieces
Lima beans	95 calories in ½ cup
Green beans	15 calories in ½ cup
Bean Sprouts	18 calories in ½ cup
Beets	30 calories in ½ cup
Broccoli	20 calories in ½ cup
Brussel sprouts	28 calories in ½ cup
Cabbage (cooked)	15 calories in ½ cup
Carrot	20 calories in 1 medium
Cauliflower	13 calories in ½ cup
Celery	5 calories in 1 stalk
Collards	27 calories in ½ cup
Corn	70 calories in 1 ear
Cucumber	30 calories in 1 medium
Lettuce	10 calories in 2 large leaves
Peas	58 calories in ½ cup
Baked potato (plain)	90 calories in 1 medium
French fries	150 calories in 10 fries (some fat)
Mashed potatoes	65 calories in ½ cup
Potato chips	115 calories in 10 chips (fatty)
Sauerkraut	22 calories in ½ cup
Spinach	20 calories in ½ cup
Zucchini	15 calories in ½ cup
Sweet potato	155 calories in 1 medium
Sweet potato (candied)	295 calories in 1 medium (some sugar)
Tomato	40 calories in 1 medium
Tofu	80 calories (low fat)

Fruits	
Apple	70 calories in 1 medium
Apple juice	120 calories in 1 cup (some sugar)
Applesauce (sweetened)	230 calories in 1 cup (some sugar)
Banana	100 calories in 1 medium (low sugar)
Blueberries	85 calories in 1 cup (low sugar)
Cantaloupe	60 calories in ½ medium (low sugar)
Fruit cocktail	195 calories in 1 cup (some sugar)
Cranapple juice	175 calories in 1 cup (some sugar)
Grapefruit	45 calories in ½ medium (low sugar)
Grapefruit juice (unsweetened)	90 calories in 1 cup
Grapes	95 calories in 1 cup (low sugar)
Grape juice	135 calories in 1 cup (some sugar)
Lemonade	110 calories in 1 cup (some sugar)
Peach	35 calories in 1 medium (low sugar)
Pear	100 calories in 1 medium (low sugar)
Pineapple (raw)	75 calories in 1 cup (low sugar)
Pineapple (canned, with syrup)	195 calories in 1 cup (sugary)
Plum	25 calories (low sugar)
Raisins	240 calories in ½ cup (sugary)
Strawberries	55 calories in 1 cup (low sugar)
Watermelon	115 calories in 1 wedge (some sugar)
Pasta, Cereals & Baked Goods	
Macaroni	190 calories in 1 cup
Macaroni and cheese	430 calories in cup (fatty)
Noodles (cooked)	200 calories in 1 cup
Rice (cooked)	110 calories in ½ cup
Spaghetti (cooked)	155 calories in 1 cup

Spaghetti with meatballs & tomato sauce	300 calories in 1 cup (some fat)
Oatmeal (cooked)	65 calories in ½ cup
Cream of wheat	100 calories in 1 cup (some sugar)
Corn flakes	100 calories in 1 cup (some sugar)
Frosted corn flakes	155 calories in 1 cup (sugary)
Shredded Wheat	90 calories in 1 biscuit
Quaker Puffed Rice	120 calories in 1 cup (some sugar)
Rice Krispies	110 calories in 1 cup (some sugar)
Special K	110 calories in 1 cup (some sugar)
Total	110 calories in 1 cup (some sugar)
Wheaties	110 calories in 1 cup (some sugar)
Cheerios	110 calories in 1 cup (some sugar)
Grape Nuts	100 calories in 1 cup
Product 19	110 calories in 1 cup (some sugar)
Bagel	165 calories in 1 (low fat)
Biscuit	105 calories in 1 (low fat)
Rye bread	60 calories in 1 slice
White bread	70 calories in 1 slice
Whole-wheat bread	65 calories in 1 slice
Hamburger or hot dog bun	120 calories in 1
Cheese pizza	185 calories in 1 medium slice (some fat)
Popcorn	40 calories in 1 cup (low fat)
Pretzel	25 calories in 1
Muffin	120 calories in 1 (low fat, low sugar)
Corn muffin	125 calories in 1 (low fat, low sugar)
Graham crackers	110 calories in 4 (low fat, low sugar)
Saltine crackers	50 calories in 4 (low fat, low sugar)
Cake doughnut (plain)	125 calories in 1 (some fat, some sugar)

Pancake (plain)	60 calories in 1 medium (low fat)
Waffle (plain)	205 calories in 1 (some fat)
Angel food cake	135 calories in 1 medium piece (some sugar)
Cupcake with icing	130 calories in 1 (some fat, sugary)
Chocolate cake	235 calories in 1 piece (some fat, sugary)
Gingerbread	175 calories in 1 piece (low fat, sugary)
Brownie	85 calories 1 medium (some fat, some sugar)
Chocolate chip cookie	50 calories 1 cookie (some fat, some sugar)
Apple pie	350 calories in 1 medium piece (fatty, sugary)
Lemon meringue pie	305 calories in 1 medium piece (fatty, sugary)
Pumpkin pie	275 calories in 1 medium piece (fatty, sugary)
Spreads, Sauces & Sweets	
Butter	35 calories in 1 pat (fatty)
Mayonnaise	100 calories in 1 tablespoon (fatty)
French salad dressing	65 calories in 1 tablespoon (fatty)
Syrup	60 calories in 1 tablespoon (sugary)
Honey	80 calories in 2 tablespoons (sugary)
Cola	145 calories in 1 can (sugary)
Fudge	115 calories in 1 ounce (some fat, sugary)
Baby Ruth	260 calories 1 bar (fatty, sugary)
Butterfingers	220 calories 1 bar (fatty, sugary)
Hershey's Milk Chocolate	190 calories 1 bar (fatty, sugary)
Hershey's Milk Chocolate with Almonds	180 calories 1 bar (fatty, sugary)
Kit Kat	180 calories 1 bar (fatty, sugary)
Kisses	28 calories 1 kiss (fatty, sugary)
Mars	235 calories 1 bar (fatty, sugary)
M & M's Plain	235 calories 1 pkg (fatty, sugary)
M & M's Peanut	240 calories 1 pkg (fatty, sugary)

Snickers	275 calories 1 bar (fatty, sugary)
Three Musketeers	255 calories 1 bar (fatty sugary)
Tootsie Roll	115 calories 1 bar (fatty, sugary)

ACTIVITY CHART
Calories Used Per Minute According to Your Weight

	Weight in Pounds		
	100	120	150
Badminton	4.3	5.2	6.5
Bicycling (slow)	3.1	3.8	4.7
Bicycling (moderate)	5.4	6.5	8.1
Calisthenics (exercises)	3.3	3.9	4.9
Cleaning windows	2.7	3.3	3.8
Conversing	1.2	1.3	1.6
Dancing, vigorous	7.8	9.1	10.0
Dressing or showering	2.1	2.6	3.2
Eating	1.1	1.3	1.5
Golf	3.6	4.3	5.4
Handball	6.3	7.6	9.5
Housework	2.7	3.1	4.0
Jogging, 11-min. mile	6.1	7.3	9.1
Mountain climbing	6.6	8.0	10.0
Mowing the grass	3.2	3.7	4.5
Running, 8-min. mile	9.4	11.3	14.1
Racquetball	6.3	7.6	9.5
School work	1.2	1.4	1.6
Shoveling snow	7.9	8.5	10.2
Skating, moderate	3.6	4.3	5.4
Skiing, downhill	6.3	7.6	9.5
Skiing, cross-country	7.2	8.7	10.8
Soccer	6.3	7.6	9.5
Sweeping the floor	2.4	2.9	3.7
Swimming, crawl stroke	5.8	6.9	8.7

Swimming, breast stroke	4.8	5.7	7.2
Table tennis	2.7	3.2	4.0
Tennis	4.5	5.4	6.8
Volleyball, moderate	2.3	2.7	3.4
Walking, slow	2.7	3.2	4.0
Walking, moderate	3.9	4.6	5.8
Watching TV	0.9	1.1	1.3

LESSON 5

GETTING IN SHAPE

In Lesson 1, you started your investigation of fitness by finding out about the who, what, when, and why of fitness. In Lesson 2, you learned about cardiovascular fitness and about exercising in your target heart-rate zone. In Lesson 3, you discovered how fit you actually are and set one or two fitness goals. Then, in Lesson 4, you learned that the balance between calories in and calories out is an important part of fitness, too. In this lesson, you get to put all of what you have learned together and start getting in shape.

READING: A TOTAL WORKOUT PLAN

Do you remember the five parts of fitness from Lesson 2: cardiovascular fitness, muscular strength, muscular endurance, flexibility, and body composition? All the parts of fitness work together to keep you looking and feeling your best.

To improve all parts of fitness, you need to develop a total workout plan. Such a plan must include activities and exercises that develop cardiovascular fitness, muscular strength, muscular endurance, and flexibility. (Body composition--your proportion of lean body mass and body fat-- follows from a combination of developing the other parts of fitness and eating nutritious foods.) The plan must develop those parts of fitness in a healthy, safe way so that you don't become injured or fatigued. That is why every workout must begin with a warm-up and end with a cool-down. Remember, fitness should be fun!

One way to set up a total workout plan is, as follows:

1.   Warm-up (flexibility) -- minimum 5 minutes (Recommended time: 10 minutes every time you exercise)

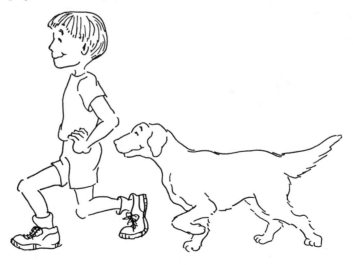

The warm-up gets you ready for more strenuous exercise. You should include stretching exercises that use all the major joints and muscles. You should use the full range of motion of each joint. Move your joints all around. As your muscles warm up, they stretch. Then, they are less likely to get injured. Stretching should be smooth, so do not bounce when you are stretching. Move from stretching to light, rhythmical exercises. Move slowly at first, gradually getting faster. The movement that warms up muscles starts the heart beating faster. As you move faster, your heart rate also will get faster. Then your heart is ready for a harder workout.

2.   Cardiovascular Fitness (aerobic activity) -- minimum 15 minutes (Recommended time: 15 to 20 minutes, three days a week)

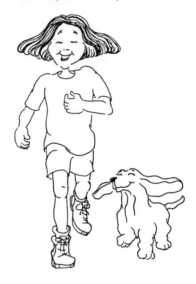

Aerobic activity improves cardiovascular fitness. In the lessons to follow, you will learn how to do some aerobic exercises that will make your heart beat faster and cause you to breathe harder. You must continue aerobic activity at an increased heart rate for at least 15 minutes each time you exercise.

3.   Muscular Strength and Endurance -- minimum 5 minutes (Recommended time: 10 minutes, 2 to 3 times a week)

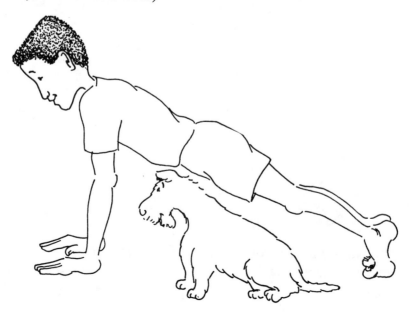

This part of the workout should provide resistance to all the major muscles of your abdomen, legs, and arms. Those exercises will help to increase strength. Do not spend too much time on one muscle group. Your breathing and heart rate should not increase too much during this part of the workout. It is not a good idea to do one exercise until you are exhausted. Instead, do a set of five to eight repetitions or "reps." Then rest. Do another set, rest, and so on. Three or four sets should be enough for each group of muscles. Remember, do not bounce or move in jerky motions. Move smoothly.

After a few days, increase the number of times you do each exercise. Continue to increase the number of times you do each exercise over many days. Once an exercise becomes easy to do ten times, make the exercise harder. Add weight, or resistance, but do the exercise fewer times. Be careful not to work your muscles so that they become sore. Sometimes, people who get sore muscles get discouraged and stop exercising.

4.   Cool-down (flexibility) -- minimum 5 minutes (Recommended time: 10 minutes every time you exercise)

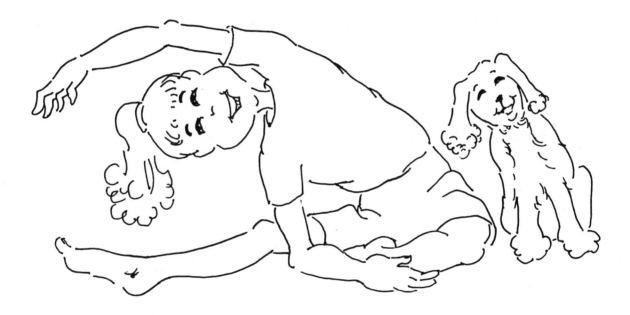

The cool-down period gives your muscles time to rebuild energy. Start by doing the aerobic exercises more slowly or by walking. Then, do some stretching, or flexibility, exercises. Now that your muscles are warmed up, they will stretch farther than they did at the beginning of the exercise period. Do stretches slowly and hold each position for a few seconds. Stretching as a cool-down exercise will help prevent soreness later. As you do your cool-down exercises, gradually slow down so your pulse rate will slow down. The cool-down period also will help you relax.

ACTIVITY: WORKING OUT

Your teacher will lead you in a complete workout that includes all components of fitness. As you go through the activities and exercises, pay attention to how you feel before, during, and after each part of the workout. During the aerobic part of the workout, remember to check every five minutes or so to see if you are exercising in your target heart-rate zone. After the workout, compare how you feel now with how you felt after the workout in Lesson 1. Do you already feel that you are getting in shape?

WRAP UP

Exercising and being active is essential for becoming physically fit. You can't get fit if you don't exercise your muscles and your heart. But, what else is part of overall fitness? What about the emotional, intellectual, and social parts of your life?

As a class, brainstorm all the other things in your life that can help you look and feel your best. (Think about your relationships with others, your approach to your school work, your extracurricular activities. How do they relate to fitness?) Write everything on a chart so you can see the list every time you come to class.

Choose one or two things you would like to change to improve your overall fitness. What help and support would you need? Don't be afraid to ask for help from your friends and family. (Don't try to do too many things at once. Working on one or two things at a time is enough.)

INVOLVING FAMILY MEMBERS

Lead a total family workout. Be sure to include a warm-up and a cool-down as part of the workout. Take turns planning fitness activities for the family. Try to plan something at least three times a week. (The plans don't have to be elaborate. Something as simple as taking a brisk walk for 15 minutes before or after dinner or walking up and down a few flights of stairs would be enough.) As the commercials used to say, "Just do it!"

LESSON 6

STRETCHING OUT

ACTIVITY: STRETCHING YOUR KNOWLEDGE

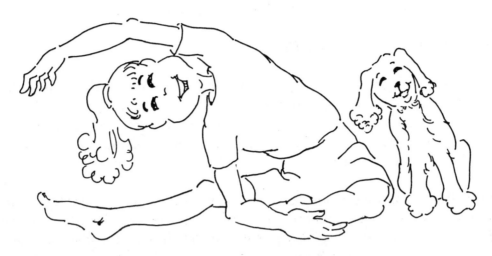

What do you know about stretching? Take this short quiz and find out.

Procedure

1. Number from 1-10 down the left side of a piece of notebook paper.
2. Read each statement that follows and decide whether the statement is true or false.
3. Write a T for true or an F for false next to the number on your paper that corresponds to the statement.
4. After you have completed all 10 statements, discuss your answers with your teacher and classmates.

TRUE OR FALSE STATEMENTS

1. The best way to stretch muscles is to bounce while you stretch.

2. Stretching is a relaxing form of exercise.

3. If you stretch after running, you will reduce the strength in your muscles.

4. You should stretch muscles after you exercise but not before you exercise.

5. Stretching should be done slowly, holding each stretch for at least 20 to 30 seconds.

6. To best increase flexibility, you should stretch as often as you can, whenever you can.

7. You can prevent injuries to your muscles by stretching.

8.   Stretch until your muscles feel a lot of tension or pull and then hold that stretch.

9.   When sitting on the floor with the legs stretched out to the sides, everyone should be flexible enough to bend forward and place his or her forehead on the floor.

10.   If you stretch too far, you will actually tighten your muscles.

READING: WHAT IS FLEXIBILITY?

An important component of fitness is **flexibility**. The root word, flexible, is defined in the dictionary as "capable of being bent, turned, or twisted without being broken." Synonyms are "pliable, elastic, resilient, springy, and supple." Think of this definition in terms of movement. What pictures come to mind? If you have ever seen a gymnast perform, you may have an idea of what flexibility of movement means.

Flexibility is a measure of how far you can move the joints and muscles in your body, such as your knees and shoulders and your back, arm, and leg muscles. Flexibility exercises improve the range of motion of the joints. Flexibility activities stretch the muscles gradually; stretched rather than tight muscles are less likely to become injured and sore. Flexibility also reduces injuries to the joints. Joint movement and stretching exercises improve flexibility and help relieve tension and stress.

Stretching is one of the best ways to improve and maintain flexibility. Stretching feels good when done correctly. Start easy and take it slowly. Try to relax. You can stretch any time you like: at school, in a car, waiting for the bus, watching TV, talking with friends, talking on the phone, reading. The best way to stretch is to spend 20 to 30 seconds in an easy stretch. Once you are relaxed, move just a little farther until you feel mild tension in your muscles. Hold that stretch a little longer. Don't bounce, and don't force yourself to stretch farther than you can comfortably. You should be able to relax while stretching.

ACTIVITY: LET'S STRETCH

Procedure

1.   Stand up and move about a little. Think about how tense or relaxed your body feels and make a mental note about how you feel.
      For example, where would you place yourself on a "tenseness" scale of 1 to 10?
      Very tense   A Little Tense   Relaxed
      1   2   3   4   5   6   7   8   9   10

2   Perform the stretches described below.
      Be sure to wear comfortable, loose-fitting clothes. Stretch only as far as your joints and muscles will allow. Don't bounce while you stretch; maintain a slow, even stretch.

3.   Stand up and move about again. How tense or relaxed does your body feel now?
      Where would you rate yourself now on the "tenseness" scale? Are you more relaxed than before?

1.   Upper Body Stretch

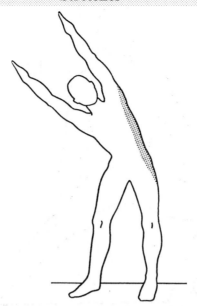

Stand erect, feet about shoulder width apart, arms raised over your head, palms facing each other. Bending at the waist, make a complete rotation of your upper body. Keep knees relaxed, not locked.

2.   The Calf Stretch

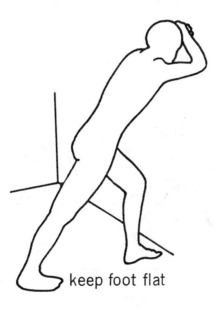

keep foot flat

Face a wall, standing 12 to 15 inches away from it. Lean against the wall, resting your forearms on the wall and your forehead on the backs of your hands. Bend one knee, moving that foot toward the wall. The back leg should be straight with the foot flat (heel down) and pointed straight ahead. Slowly move your hips forward, still keeping the back leg straight and foot flat. Create an easy stretch in your calf muscle and hold for 20 to 30 seconds. Now stretch the other calf muscle.

The stretching activities were excerpted from *STRETCHING*© 1980
by Bob & Jean Anderson. Shelter Publications, Bolinas, CA.
Distributed in bookstores by Random House, Reprinted by permission.
For a free catalog of Stretching Inc. products/publications contact:
Stretching, Inc. P. O. Box 767, Palmer Lake, CO 80133
or call 800-333-1307.
43

3.   Side Lunge

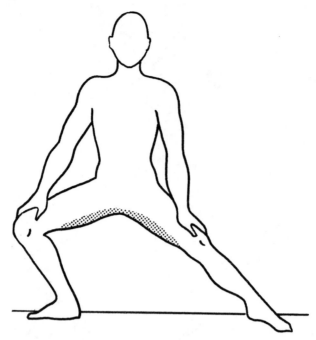

Stand erect, feet parallel and shoulder width apart. Turn your right foot to the right so it is at a right angle to your left foot. Take a long step to your right. Hold for 10-20 seconds. Return to a standing position, turn left foot and lunge to your left. Hold for 10-20 seconds. Repeat to each side.

4.   Hamstring and Ankle Stretch

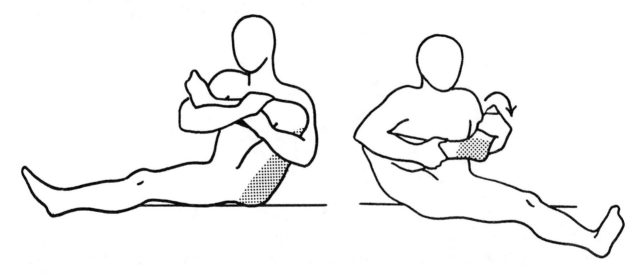

Sit with your legs straight out in front of you. Bend one knee toward your chest. Hold onto the outside of that ankle with one hand and place your other hand and forearm around your bent knee. Gently pull the leg as one unit toward your chest until you feel an easy stretch in the back of the leg. Hold for 20 seconds. (Make sure there is no pull or stress on the knee.) Lessen the stretch a little and use the hand around the ankle to rotate your ankle clockwise and then counter-clockwise through a complete range of motion. Repeat 10 to 20 times in each direction. Repeat with the other leg and ankle.

5.   The Spinal Twist

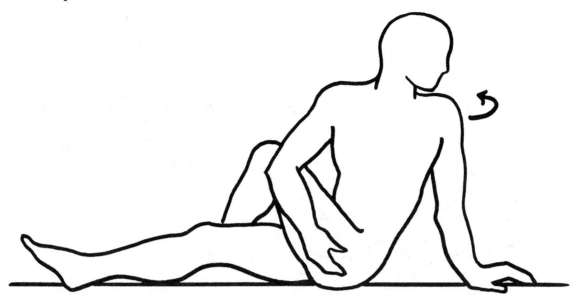

Sit with the right leg straight. Bend your left leg, cross your left foot over and rest it to the outside of your right knee. Then, bend your right elbow and rest it on the outside of your upper left thigh, just above the knee. With your left hand resting behind you, slowly turn your head to look over your left shoulder and, at the same time, rotate your upper body toward your left hand and arm. As you rotate your body, push the right elbow against the left knee to keep the left leg stationary. You should feel this stretch in your upper back, lower back, side, and upper leg. Hold for 15 seconds. Repeat on the other side.

6.   Shoulder and Arm Stretch

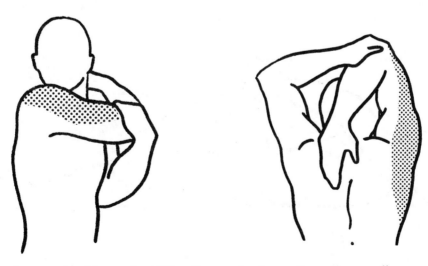

To stretch your shoulder and middle of upper back, gently pull your elbow across your chest toward your opposite shoulder. Keep your elbow slightly lower than your shoulder. Hold for 10 seconds. Then, with arms overhead, hold the elbow of that arm with the hand of the other arm. Gently pull the elbow behind your head, creating a stretch in the upper arm and side. Hold for 15 seconds. Repeat both stretches with the other arm.

7. Groin Stretch

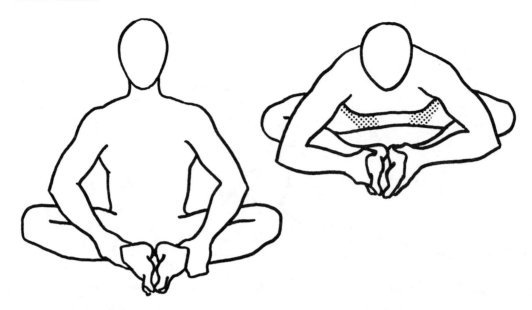

Sit on the floor with the soles of your feet together. Put your hands around your feet so that your elbows are slightly in front of your lower legs. Gently pull your body forward until you feel a stretch in your inner thigh (groin) area. Keep your lower back flat; do not bend your head down toward your hands. Face forward. Increase the stretch until you feel tension but not pain. Hold the stretch for 30 seconds and concentrate on how your muscles feel. Release the stretch slowly.

8. Quadriceps Stretch

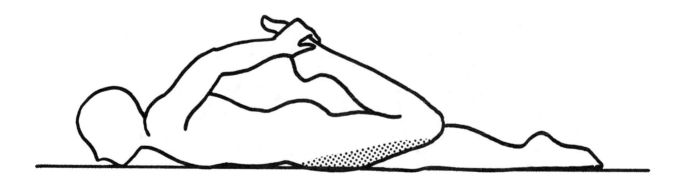

Lie on stomach with head down. With right hand pull right foot toward the buttocks. Hold for 15 to 30 seconds. Repeat with left leg. You should feel the stretch in the quadricep muscle, the large muscle at the front of the thigh.

9.   Lower Back Stretch

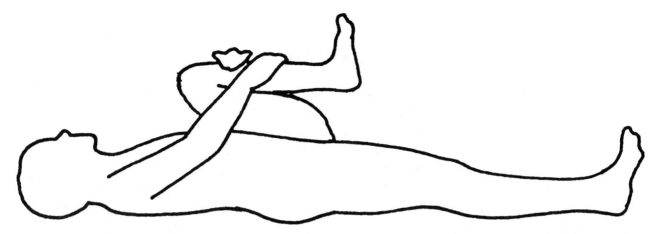

Lie on your back. Bend one knee toward your chest. Grasp your leg just below the knee and gently pull your knee toward your chest. You should feel a stretch in the back of your leg. Keep your lower back pressed into the floor while you stretch. Hold the stretch for 30 seconds. Release slowly and stretch the other leg.

As a variation, stretch the outside of your leg by pulling the bent leg slightly toward the opposite shoulder. Keep your back flat on the floor. Hold for 20 seconds. Do both legs, one at a time.

Stretch both legs by bringing both knees into the chest. First keep your head down, then curl your head up toward your knees and hold that position. Then, straighten out your legs and arms and relax.

10.   Whole Body Stretch

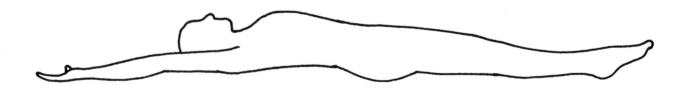

Lie on your back with your arms straight over your head and legs extended straight in front. Stretch arms and legs (point the toes) feeling as though you are making your body longer. Pull in your abdominal muscles to make the middle of your body thin and press the small of your back into the floor. Hold this stretch for five seconds. Release. Repeat the stretch three times. This stretch is good for your arms, shoulders, spine, abdominal muscles, legs, feet, and ankles.

WRAP UP

Work with a partner and outline a stretching plan that you might use every day. List the stretches you would include in your plan. Make sure that you have included stretches for all parts of your body, especially your legs, arms, and back. Describe the stretches you would include and draw diagrams of those stretches. You might compile your descriptions and drawings into a booklet that you can keep in your room as a reminder to stretch when you get up and before you go to bed.

INVOLVING FAMILY MEMBERS

Give family members the quiz that began this lesson. How much do they know about stretching? Then, lead family members in a stretching session as a warm-up to an aerobic activity such as basketball, walking, or bicycling. Make sure you stretch out your muscles after the activity, too.

LESSON 7

MUSCULAR STRENGTH AND ENDURANCE

READING: ASK MR. MUSCLES

How much do you know about muscular strength and endurance? If you're not sure, just ask Mr. Muscles!

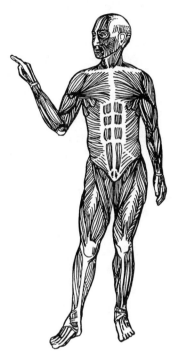

Q: What does my age have to do with my muscles?

A: *Most people can't really change their muscles much until they're teenagers. At puberty, our bodies go through the physical changes that turn us into adults. One of the hormones (body chemicals) that causes these changes is testosterone, which affects muscle development. Boys can take much longer to go through puberty than girls, but by the late teens most should have enough testosterone to bring about muscle changes.*

Q: Do some people have more muscles than others?

A: *We are all born with the same basic muscles—Arnold Schwarzenegger, Pee Wee Herman, and you. Why don't your muscles look quite like Arnold's? You can blame (or thank) your age, sex, and parents, as well as your exercise patterns. These four things influence the size and shape of your major muscles.*

Q: Why aren't girls and boys alike when it comes to muscles?

A: *Females have much less testosterone, the hormone needed for muscle-building. That's why they can develop hard, strong muscles, but will never build big ones, no matter how much they exercise. Compare the powerful yet slim legs of a ballerina to the powerful yet bulging ones of a football player. Both have strong muscles, but a very different shape.*

49

Q: Does the exercise I do affect the shape and size of my muscles?

A: *Yes. Most popular sports and exercises will give you strong muscles, not bulging ones. Developing big muscles requires a special kind of training, called progressive overload. Muscle-builders train with a weight so heavy they can lift it only 8 to 12 times. They gradually move up to even heavier weights. Over-stressing the muscle repeatedly creates little tears in it. When the body repairs those tears, the muscle gets bigger. A different kind of training builds hard but not big muscles. You train with less weight, but lift it many times—40 or 50 times or more. You don't move on to heavier weights.*

Q: What else affects the size and shape of my muscles?

A: *Like the color of your eyes and hair, your basic body shape and muscle tissue are inherited from your parents. Every exerciser can work on his or her muscular appearance and strength, but results will differ from person to person. Some people can train very hard but their muscles will never be big. Others can build bulging ones with much less effort.*

Q: Is muscle-building a good idea for kids?

A: *Most famous bodybuilders didn't start serious training until their late teens. They followed strict training programs designed to build muscles slowly without injury. Too many teenagers take risks by using weights at home with little or no coaching.*

Q: Will big muscles make me a better athlete?

A: *Not necessarily. Big muscles are usually strong muscles. Pure strength is important in sports like football and wrestling. Soccer, swimming, track, basketball, tennis, karate, and many other sports rely more on skill, speed, agility, and stamina than simple muscle power. Spending all your training time on building big arm, chest, and leg muscles usually isn't the best way to improve your overall performance. In general, coaches say that the best training for a sport is playing that sport. You'll gain skill while you exercise the exact muscles for the action.*

Q: What is the best training program for kids?

A.   *A program that leads to overall fitness is best. Aim for 30 minutes of exercise every other day. Choose activities that get your heart pounding and your lungs panting. You'll develop a strong heart, powerful lungs, and many efficient muscles rather than just a few large ones.*

ACTIVITY: BECOMING STRONGER

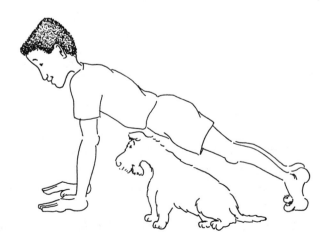

Procedure

1. Read the exercising tips that follow. Discuss their importance with your teacher and classmates.

Exercising Do's and Don'ts

- Perform conditioning exercises carefully and with control. Rapid repetitions are not safe.
- Do not hold your breath while you exercise. Practice good breathing techniques by exhaling when you are contracting your muscles.
- Use a mat or carpeted surface for floor exercises.
- Make sure you are not arching your back during the exercises. During floor exercises, keep your lower back flat or pressed into the floor or mat at all times.
- Perform repetitions until you feel the muscles fatiguing. Then, do a few more repetitions, but do not push yourself to the point of pain. Pain can mean injury.
- Be sensible if you use weights. You should be able to complete a set of 10 to 12 repetitions without stopping. If you are unable to complete 10 repetitions, then you are probably using too much weight.
- Follow these general guidelines:

  Beginner -- 1 set of 10 to 12 repetitions

  Intermediate -- 2 sets of 10 to 12 repetitions

  Advanced -- 3 sets of 10 to 12 repetitions

Work up from one level to the next. Do not assume you are ready for the advanced stage until you have successfully completed the other two.

---

2. Warm up before you begin the exercises for muscular strength.
    You might stretch or walk around the room. Try to relax and stretch out all parts of your body--your legs, your arms, your back, your shoulders, and your abdomen. Take your joints through their full range of motion.

3. Perform the exercises that follow for muscular strength.
    If you have not exercised much lately, your muscles will be out of shape. Start easy and remember that this is not a competition to see who can do more repetitions. When you become tired or your muscles feel sore, stop. You can injure your muscles or joints if you work too hard before you are ready.

4. Stretch out the muscles that you worked during this session.
    You might use some of the stretches from the previous lesson.

5. Make a note of which exercises were easy for you to do and which were difficult.
    For exercises that were difficult, indicate which of your major muscle groups need the most work. Those are the areas that you should concentrate on with a gradual increase in exercises that work those areas.

6. Read the information that follows about specificity and overload.
    The information should help you decide which muscles to work on and how to make them stronger without injury.

Exercises for Strong Abdominal (Stomach) Muscles   (from easy to more difficult)

1.   Pelvic Tilt

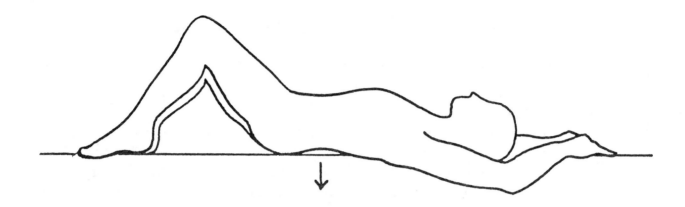

Lie on your back with your knees bent and feet flat on the floor, slightly apart. Press the lower part of your back down to the floor by contracting your abdominal and gluteal (buttocks) muscles. Hold the contraction for about five seconds. The lumbar spine (lower portion of the spine) should be pressed firmly against the mat or floor. Release and repeat.

2.   Abdominal Curls

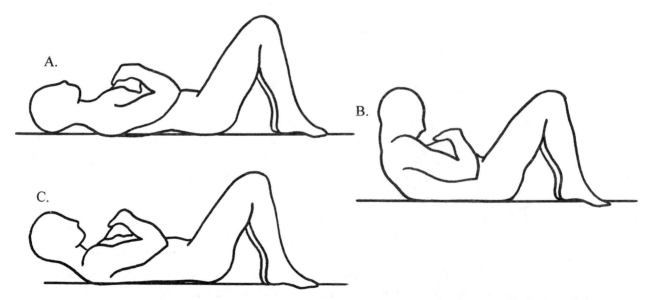

Lie on your back with your knees bent, feet flat on the floor, hands across your chest (A). Relax your neck and shoulders. Curl upper body forward and up until your shoulders lift from the floor (B). Hold for 5 seconds and return the upper body to the floor (C). Tighten your upper abdominal muscles as you curl up. Rest for 5 seconds and repeat.

3. Elbow to Knee Abdominal Curls

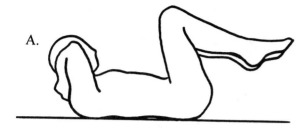

A.

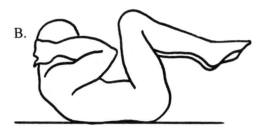

B.

Start in the same position as for abdominal curls. Place your fingertips behind your head, but do not lace your fingers together. (Your fingertips should support your head, but not pull up on your neck.) Raise your feet off the floor (A). Using your abdominal muscles, hold your upper body at about a 30-degree angle off the floor. Then, bring your elbows forward and try to touch your thighs about 1-2 inches above the knee (B). Uncurl and return your upper body to the floor (A). Repeat. Be sure to keep your lower back flat and pushed into the floor or mat during abdominal exercises.

4. Abdominal Obliques

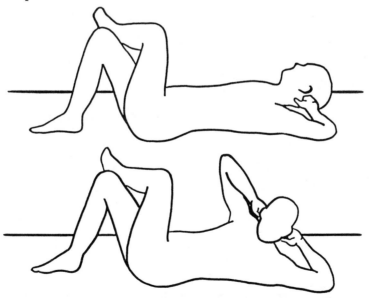

Lie on back with right leg bent and opposite leg crossed over the knee. Place hands behind head with fingertips just behind ears. Slowly twist the torso bringing the right shoulder toward the left knee of the crossed leg. Do not pull on your head neck to lift yourself; use your abdominal muscles. Repeat the same movement on the other side.

5.   Advanced Upper Abdominal Curls

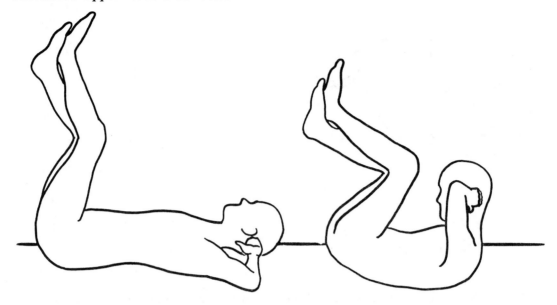

Lie on your back with your legs elevated into the air and ankles crossed. Hold hands behind head with fingertips just behind ears. Keep your lower back pressed into the floor. Draw your knees toward your chest as you curl your upper body forward.

Exercises for Strong Legs and Buttocks   (from easy to more difficult)

1.   Leg Lifts

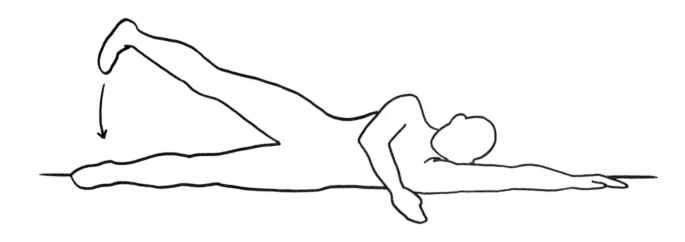

Lie on one side with head resting on shoulder, lower arm extended. Lift top leg to about a 45 degree angle and gradually lower it. (Lower leg can be bent or straight.) Muscles get the best workout when toes of upper leg are turned downward to that toes touch heel of lower foot when leg is lowered. Move leg slowly up and down; don't let gravity take over on way down, but control the downward movement. Repeat with other leg.

2.   Cross Leg Lifts

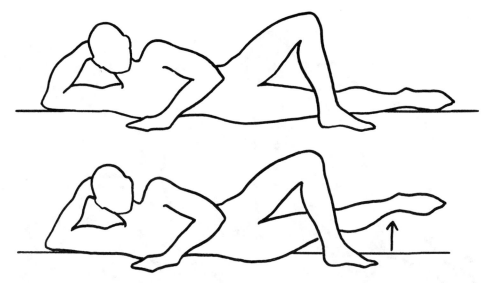

Lie on one side with legs straight. Prop yourself up on your elbow with head resting on hand, other arm in front, palm on floor for balance. Bend your top leg and place that foot on the floor just in front of your bottom knee. While in that position, raise and lower your bottom leg. Switch side.

3.   Outer Thigh

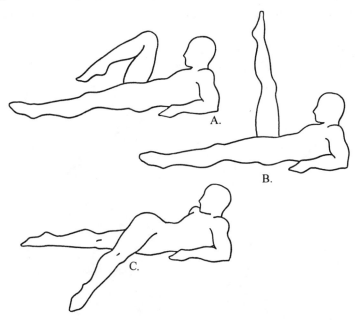

A.

B.

C.

Lie on back, legs out straight, and lift yourself onto your elbows. Bend your right knee into your chest (A). Then, straighten leg and point toe toward ceiling (B). With a controlled motion, lower your right leg (still straight) over your left leg at a right angle (C). Lift the right leg back to position B, bend knee (A), and return leg to floor. Repeat and then change legs.

4.   Doggie

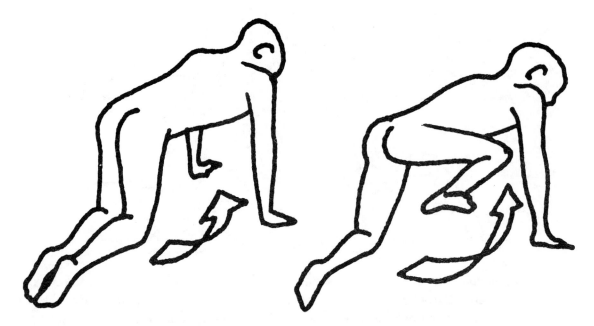

Balance on hands and knees keeping head straight forward and back level or slightly rounded. (Do not let back arch.) Lift right leg to side with knee bent. Leg forms a right angle to body when lifted. Lower leg and repeat. Repeat with other leg. Be sure body stays straight; do not rock or lean to the side. Tighten buttocks as you lift leg.

5.   Half-knee Bends

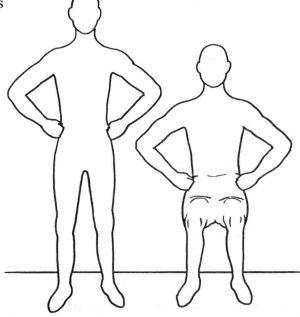

Stand with feet shoulder-width apart. Place hands on hips or straight out in front of body. Squat until the thighs are parallel to the floor and then return to a standing position. Repeat. (Do not bend all the way down; full-knee bends put too much pressure on the knees.)

1.   Arm Circles

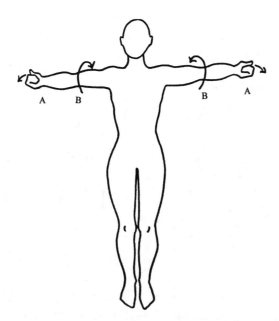

In standing position, hold arms straight out at shoulder level, palms facing ceiling. Make fists and move arms in small circles going forward. Change directions and make circles going backward. Gradually make circles larger and rotate through shoulder joint. Gradually make circles smaller again.

2.   Coffee Grinder

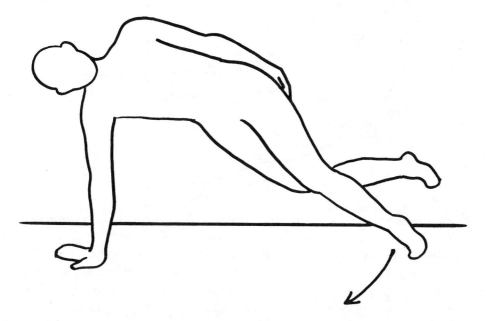

Lie on your right side. Lift yourself up on your right arm keeping both feet on the floor. Keeping your right arm fully extended and your legs straight, "walk" your body in a complete circle using your right arm as a pivot. Repeat. Then, change arms.

3.   Reverse Push-ups

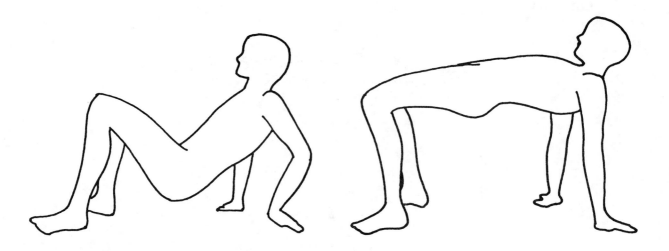

Assume crab position facing toward ceiling. Palms and feet are flat on the floor, knees and elbows are bent. Raise and lower body by bending at the elbows. Look at your knees as you do this exercise. Raise your hips as high as you can off the floor when you straighten your arms. Repeat.

4.   Modified Pull-ups

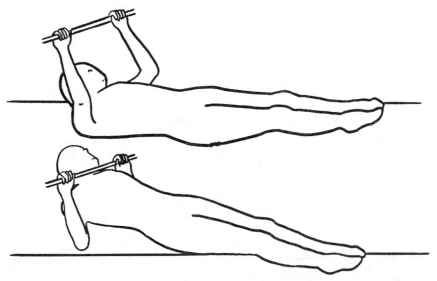

Place a strong pole or pipe on the seats of two chairs placed about 4 feet apart. Make sure the ends of the bar and the chairs are secure. Lie on your back, slide under the bar and grasp it with two hands, palms facing away from your body and hands about shoulder-width apart. Pull your chest up to the bar keeping your body straight from head to feet. Repeat. (If this is too easy, then find a higher bar. This is a good exercise to train for the chin-up task. Gradually move to the horizontal chin-up bar.)

5.   Push-ups

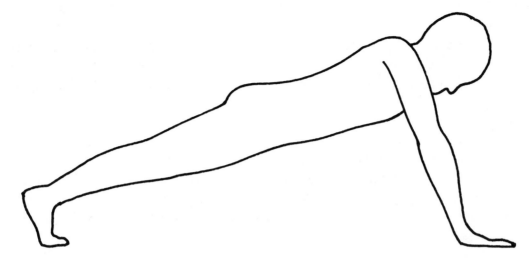

One of the best exercises for increasing upper body strength is the push-up. Lie on your stomach with your hands on either side of your shoulders. (Elbows will be bent.) Push body up with arms until arms are straight. You can use either your toes or knees as the contact point with the floor. (Push-ups from the knees are easier than push-ups from the toes.) Lower body so that nose nearly touches the floor; do not let chest touch the floor. As you raise and lower body, keep body in a straight line with back flat.

READING: SPECIFICITY AND OVERLOAD

To be physically fit, you need strong muscles. Those muscles don't have to be as strong as a bodybuilder's muscles; they just have to be strong enough to allow you to move easily in all directions without injuring yourself. Muscular strength and endurance are part of the important components of overall fitness.

There are two ideas about strengthening your muscles that you should understand before you begin an exercise program. One is **specificity** and the other is **overload**. Specificity is pretty simple. It means that only specific exercises will strengthen specific muscles. In other words, abdominal curls or crunches will make your stomach muscles stronger, but they won't do a thing for your thighs. Chin-ups or push-ups will make your arms stronger, but they still won't get at those thighs. You have to do the specific exercises that make particular muscles stronger. If you want to improve your performance on the chin-ups task, for example, then you must perform exercises that use and strengthen the muscles in your upper body.

Overload is a bit harder to figure out because it will be different for each person. Basically, overload means that your muscles will not become stronger unless you exercise them at a higher-than-normal level. You have to push your muscles a little beyond what they can already do. Once your muscles are stronger through exercise, the exercises will become easier and you can move from the beginner to the intermediate level. The secret is to know your own body and to work at a level that is best for you.

In developing muscular strength and endurance, concentrate mainly on three muscle groups: the abdominal (stomach) muscles, the muscles of the legs and buttocks, and the muscles of the upper body (arms, chest, and shoulders). Notice that the exercises you performed in this lesson were divided into those three specific groups. Usually, some muscle groups are stronger than others. This will vary from person to person. You should work all three muscle groups, but especially those that are weak. Remember, start easy with weak muscles. You must strengthen them gradually over time to avoid injury.

Remember, if you are worried about developing bulging muscles, doing these types of exercises for muscular strength and endurance won't make your muscles bulge. You must go through very specialized training programs to build big muscles like Arnold Schwarzenegger's. Exercises for muscular strength will make your muscles stronger, keep your skin looking healthier and less baggy, and will give definition to your arms, legs, and abdomen. You will just look better, not muscle-bound.

Muscular endurance is also an important part of developing strong muscles. Endurance is the ability of the muscles to do the same motion over and over again for increasing periods of time. When you have muscular endurance, you can work and play for a long time and your muscles will not get tired. The number of curl-ups or pull-ups you can do is related to your muscular endurance and your muscular strength. How long you can shovel snow, hit a tennis ball, wash windows, or jog is due to your muscular (and cardiovascular) endurance, not just strength.

Stop and Discuss

1. Describe exercises that are specific to the upper body, the abdomen, and the legs and buttocks. Explain the principle of specificity as it relates to those exercises.
2. How will you know if you are applying the principle of overload appropriately?
3. What are the benefits of developing muscular strength and endurance?
4. How might you improve muscular strength and endurance during daily activities?

WRAP UP

Read the following information about steroids. What do you think about the use of steroids to build muscular strength in amateur and professional athletes?

"Muscle" drugs, known as steroids, cause many problems for the athletes who use them. Some have died of cancer, and others have serious physical ailments including liver damage. Sports competitors have lost their Olympic medals when steroids showed up in their urine tests. Increased use by young people has caused even more worry.

Users hope these artificial hormones will quickly increase their muscle size and weight, but the drugs have some scary side effects. Female users may develop beards or lose their menstrual periods. Males may become overly aggressive or develop breasts. Steroid use can lead to serious liver problems. If taken before you reach your full height, they can stunt your growth.

Users who take steroids without medical advice may know little about the side effects. They see the drugs as an aid to winning a place on the school team. They don't fully realize the serious risks they're taking with their bodies.

But the experts agree—steroids and sports don't mix. There are no short cuts to becoming a trained athlete.

Find out more about steroids. Why is their use banned from amateur athletic competitions? What are the side effects? How long before the side effects occur? Are the short-term results worth the long-term risks?

INVOLVING FAMILY MEMBERS

Lead your family members in a 10-minute workout to develop muscular strength. Include the exercises you did in class or find a book of exercises that develop muscular strength in the abdomen, legs, and upper body. (If you use exercises from a book, let your teacher review the exercises before you use them to make sure they are safe and will not hurt someone's back or joints.) Tell your family members what you learned about specificity and overload as you do the exercises together.

Perform exercises for muscular strength at least three times a week. You can do these exercises easily while watching television. Plan one or two exercises for each commercial break.

SPORTS, PHYSICAL ACTIVITIES, AND FITNESS

Three activity patterns are related to how fit American children and teenagers are

- year-round physical activity,
- exposure to a wide variety of activities through physical education class at school, and
- participation in a variety of physical activities outside of school.

How do your personal activity patterns measure up?

ACTIVITY: MY ACTIVITY PATTERNS

How much time do you spend each week in physical activities? Do you think it is a lot of time, a reasonable amount of time, or very little time? Take this personal survey and compare the time you spend doing various activities.

Procedure

1. Copy the following data table, How I Usually Spend My Time, onto a sheet of notebook paper.
   You can save time by writing only the key words in the activity column, such as school, PE, sleep, TV, housework, friends, and so on.
2. Complete the data table by estimating the number of hours (or portions of hours) you spend doing each activity on a "typical" weekday and on a "typical" weekend day.
   Of course, your activity patterns change from day to day, but think about what you usually do on weekdays and on weekends. Make sure the total hours for one day are not more than 24.
3. Think about your answers to the Stop and Discuss questions that follow the data table. Discuss your answers with your classmates.

How I Usually Spend My Time

Activity		Weekday	Saturday or Sunday
1.	I am in school for	__ hours	__ hours
2.	I am in physical education class for	__ hours	__ hours
3.	I usually sleep for	__ hours	__ hours
4.	I usually watch TV for	__ hours	__ hours
5.	I help at home (yardwork, cleaning, washing dishes) for	__ hours	__ hours
6.	I am with or talk to my friends for	__ hours	__ hours
7.	I interact with family members for	__ hours	__ hours
8.	I am involved in some type of physical activity (exercise, sports, games) for	__ hours	__ hours
9.	I do homework for	__ hours	__ hours
10.	I work at a job outside of school for	__ hours	__ hours
11.	Other ways I spend my time:		
	a. _____	__ hours	__ hours
	b. _____	__ hours	__ hours
	c. _____	__ hours	__ hours

LESSON 9

QUACKERY DETECTION

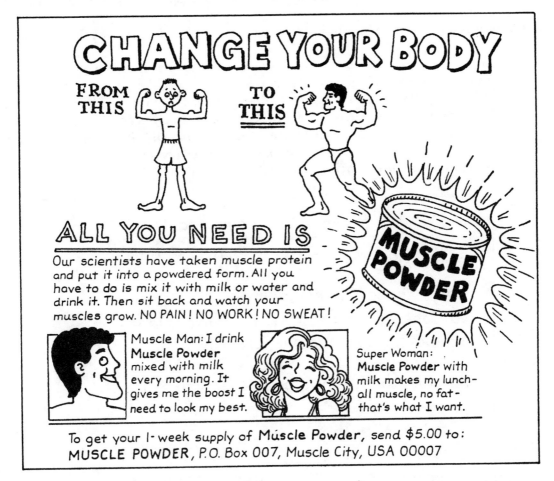

Would you believe this ad for Muscle Powder? Why or why not? Do you know anyone who might order Muscle Powder or something similar? Why do some people fall for scams that promise a more perfect body but that don't have much chance of working?

False and misleading ads, such as the one for Muscle Powder, are examples of quackery. A quack is a person who falsely claims to have certain medical skills. Quackery includes anything a quack does to treat people. It also includes advertising products or treatments that do not do what they claim to do. Sometimes, the products or treatments are even dangerous.

The ad for Muscle Powder was for a product. The other ads in this lesson are for treatments or services. Do you know enough about fitness to avoid being taken in by such ads? Find out in the next activity.

ACTIVITY: TRUTH IN ADVERTISING

In this activity, you will decide which fitness club is likely to help you become fit and which might take you for a ride. To make your decision, you must collect evidence from the ads. It pays to read carefully and to become a wise consumer.

Procedure

1. Read the advertisements that follow for the Springs Wellness Spa and the Fizz-eek Fitness Center.
2. Write the evidence from each ad that supports or does not support the claim that you can become fit by joining.
3. Decide which fitness club you would join and write the name of the spa or the fitness center on your paper.
   You can decide to join both clubs or to join neither club. Be prepared to support your decision with your evidence from Step 2.
4. Pretend that you will visit both the Springs Wellness Spa and the Fizz-eek Fitness Center. Write a list of questions that you would want someone to answer before you decided to join.
   Think about what you have learned about fitness throughout this unit. What would you need to know about the services of each fitness club to decide if you could become more fit?
5. Discuss your decision and list of questions with your teacher and classmates.

Springs Wellness Spa

Join <u>now</u> during our SPRING FLING!

Get in shape for the summer and take advantage of our 2-for-1 special. You and a friend can join for one low rate. *

For your body-shaping needs, you can choose from our
- whirlpool baths
- saunas
- massages
- free weights
- mud wraps
- mineral water soaks
- tanning beds
- aerobics classes

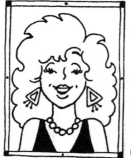

Our founder, Lita Lepke, studied in the great spas of Europe and trained all our personnel in these world-famous procedures. You would have to spend thousands of dollars to get these same treatments in the European spas. Call to find out about our low monthly payment schedule.

Why wait? Start creating a new you today!
Call 555-8769 for your first appointment.

* Applies only to yearly memberships.

Fizz-eek Fitness Center

Stop by our center at 10 First Street for a tour and receive one week's membership **FREE**. Once you have seen what we have to offer, you'll want to come back for more!

Members receive fitness testing the first week. We check progress regularly. An exercise physiologist consults with each member to set up a **fitness** program tailored to meet that member's personal goals.

Our equipment includes

- exercycles (bikes)
- indoor track
- universal weights
- rowing machines
- swimming pool
- cross-country ski tracks

We have aerobics, low-impact aerobics, and swimming classes for pre-schoolers through seniors. The whole family can get in shape and have fun together.

Trained physical educators lead all our classes and provide help to members working out on their own. With their doctor's permission, even people with health problems can participate. We will work with your doctor and design a special program for you.

CALL 555-5647 today for your tour
Or stop by between 7 a.m. and 10 p.m.

WRAP UP

You can avoid the fitness quacks by becoming a wise consumer of fitness and nutritional products. Find advertisements in the newspaper or in magazines for fitness equipment, services, or products and bring those ads to class. Working with a partner or in teams, examine the claims the ads make and decide whether you believe the claims. Remember to look for evidence that supports the claims. Determine what else you would need to know about the product, service, or equipment before you spend your money.

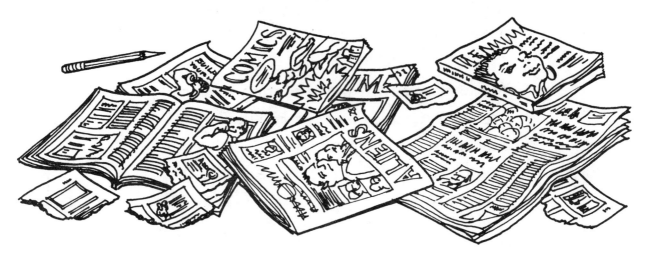

Share the ads your team examined. Discuss the evidence you used to decide whether the service or equipment would do what the ad claims. Post the ads on chart paper or on a bulletin board under appropriate headings, such as "Look at the Quacks We Found" and "We Can Buy These Ads." Discuss what else you would need to know before actually purchasing the equipment, products, or services. How could you find out what you need to know?

Examine the posted ads. Does everyone agree with the placement of the ads? Why might there be differences of opinion? What else could you do to become physically fit rather than spending your money on the advertised product, service, or equipment?

INVOLVING FAMILY MEMBERS

Help your family members become "quackery detectives." Find ads for fitness equipment, services, or other products that claim to give you the perfect body. Examine the ads with your family members and discuss why some family members might buy the product and others would not. Look for evidence that the claims are legitimate and not from a "quack." Work at becoming wise consumers so you will not be taken in by false advertising claims.

FITNESS PLANNING

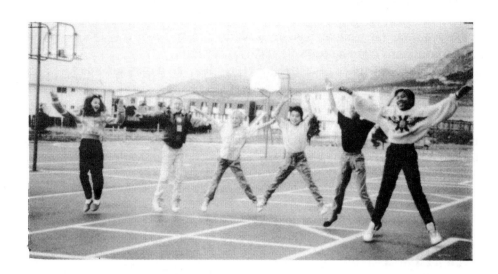

When was the last time you were involved in a physical activity that really made you work, one that made you sweat and breathe hard? Do all of the activities you participate in make you sweat and breathe hard? By now, you know that to become physically fit you need to exercise three to four times a week for 15-20 minutes at your target heart rate. To exercise at that level, you will need to choose activities that will increase your heart rate and make you sweat and breathe hard.

These same physical fitness activities affect your health in many ways. People who exercise regularly report that they feel better, have more energy, and often require less sleep. Regular exercisers often lose excess weight and improve their muscular strength, flexibility, and cardiovascular efficiency.

Despite knowing all the benefits of exercise, most people do not exercise often or vigorously enough to achieve maximum health benefits. It becomes easier to sit in front of the television, but watching television is not as much fun as getting out there and doing something!

In this lesson, you will plan a two-week fitness program and talk about what will help you stick to it. The fitness habits you start now could last a lifetime.

ACTIVITY: PUT YOUR BODY IN MOTION

Before you develop a plan, you should review the components of a complete workout and what it feels like to exercise at your target heart rate. You and your classmates will plan this workout. This is your chance to make working out motivating and FUN!
Procedure

1.   Your teacher will assign you and your partner or teammates one component of fitness: warm-up exercises, cardiovascular fitness, muscular strength and endurance, or cool-down (flexibility).

2. Review the lesson or lessons in this unit that will help you plan activities for your assigned part of the workout.

   For example, if your team is responsible for muscular strength and endurance, then you should review Lesson 7.

3. Prepare to lead the class in the activities or exercises you suggested for your assigned component of fitness.

   Decide who will demonstrate each exercise or activity you chose. Be sure your teacher approves your plan.

4. Participate in a complete workout plan designed by you and your classmates. Be sure you begin with the warm-up activities and end with the cool down.

5. Discuss the activities you liked best. Could you do those activities at home?

ACTIVITY: DEVELOPING A PERSONAL FITNESS PLAN

Now that you and your teammates have reviewed what goes into a fitness plan, it's time for you to make one. This needs to be a personal plan, one that you can follow. It should have all the components of fitness, but be organized in a way that is right for you.

Procedure

1. Review your list from the Wrap Up of Lesson 8 of the activities you like to do. As you look over the activities, ask yourself these questions:

   a. Have I included activities that will improve all parts of fitness--cardiovascular fitness, muscular strength, muscular endurance, and flexibility?

   b. Have I included activities that will make my heart beat faster for at least 15 minutes?

   c. Have I chosen activities I really like to do?

   d. Have I involved my friends or my family in my activities?

2. Make two fitness charts like the one shown below.

   Remember, you need to make a two-week plan. One week might not be long enough for you to figure out what you like to do and how to build exercise into your schedule.

MY FITNESS PLAN

Day	Warm-up Activities	Aerobic Activities	Strength Activities	Cool-down Activities	When?	Where?	With Whom?

3. Complete the first column of the chart by writing which activity (or activities) you plan to do on each day of the week.

   Set realistic goals for YOU. Don't set goals based on what you think someone would expect you to do. Which activities will you really be likely to do? You may list an activity more than once.

4.   Next, write **when** you will exercise, **where** you will exercise, and **with whom**.
     You may work with a partner to complete your fitness chart. You can suggest activities or exercises to one another. You can help one another decide when you would be likely to exercise, where, and with whom. It is important to make a complete plan because you will be more likely to stick to it if you involve other people and know where and when you will exercise.

5.   Look at your list again. Below your list or on the back of the paper, write what would keep you from doing these activities. Leave a space or two between each reason for not exercising or being active.
     Your reasons could be things such as, "I don't look good in exercise clothes. I think other kids would laugh or make fun of me behind my back." Or, "It costs money to go skating and I never have enough money." Or, "My best friend is really into jogging, but I hate jogging."

6.   After each reason for not doing an activity, write something that could motivate you to do the activity.
     Your motivators could be things such as, "I could just wear baggy pants and a T-shirt and not worry about special exercise clothes." Or, "If I did a couple more chores at home, then my parents might raise my allowance and I would have money to go skating." Or, "I like riding my bike around. I guess I could ask someone else to go bike riding." Try to be realistic about your motivators, but try to get rid of your excuses for not exercising.

7.   Once you have filled in all the boxes, look over one another's fitness plans and identify ways to help one another succeed.
     If you want to do some activities that you are unable to do, ask your partner for help. Maybe together you can figure out ways to help you overcome the problems. Sometimes, people get discouraged after a short time because they do not see any changes. Think of ways you and your partner can encourage each other if one of you gets discouraged.

8.   Show your chart to your teacher for approval.

9.   As a class, decide how you could reward one another for following your plans.

WRAP UP

Check in with your classmates every day during the week. Find out which of you followed your fitness plans the previous day. Congratulate those who did. Encourage those who had problems or are giving up, and help one another find ways to overcome any problems. Try to get everyone to continue with their plans.

Talk about any changes you decided to make in your fitness plans. Did you find activities that you like better? Did a friend invite you to do something that was more fun than what you had in your plan?

Discuss the results of your fitness activities. Do you feel better after exercising? Do you think you will become more active on a regular basis? Why or why not?

Your fitness level probably will not change in just one or two weeks, but trying to set aside time for fitness will help you change your life for lifelong fitness. If you keep with it, you will notice changes in how you feel and how you look. Keep up the good work!

INVOLVING FAMILY MEMBERS

Make a fitness plan as a family. What activities could you do together? You might make plans to do something simple like walking together or you could plan more elaborate activities like going on hikes or participating on community teams through the parks and recreation department. The important goal is to get off the couch, turn off the television, and get moving! Even if you are active for only 20 to 30 minutes each day, you will be on your way to feeling good and looking good.

DATE DUE

GAYLORD			PRINTED IN U.S.A.